LUXURIOUS LOVING

LUXURIOUS LOVING

Tantric Inspirations for Passion and Pleasure

Barbara Carrellas

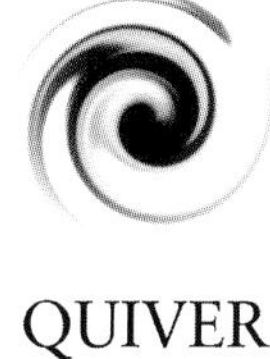

QUIVER

First published in the USA in 2006 by
Quiver, a member of
Quayside Publishing Group
33 Commercial Street
Gloucester, MA 01930

The publisher maintains the records relating to images in this book required by 18 USC 2257, which records are located at Rockport Publishers, Inc., 33 Commercial Street, Gloucester, MA 01930.

10 09 08 07 06 1 2 3 4 5

ISBN - 13: 978-1-59233-237-3
ISBN - 10: 1-59233-237-4

Library of Congress Cataloging-in-Publication Data available

Cover design by Michael Brock
Book design by Laura Herrmann Design
Photography by Allan Penn
Female model: April Blossom

DEDICATION

for Kate with love

TABLE OF CONTENTS

Contents

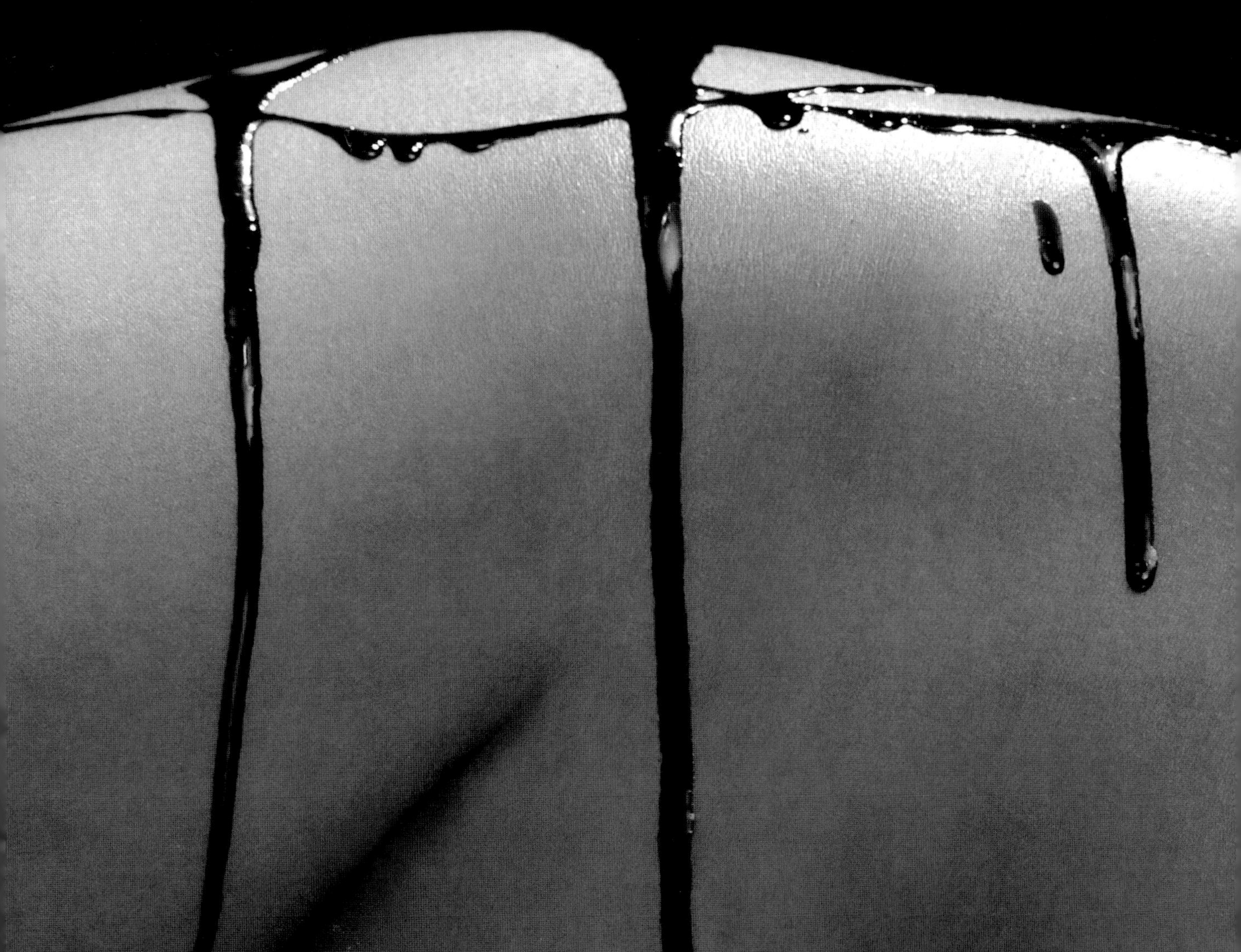

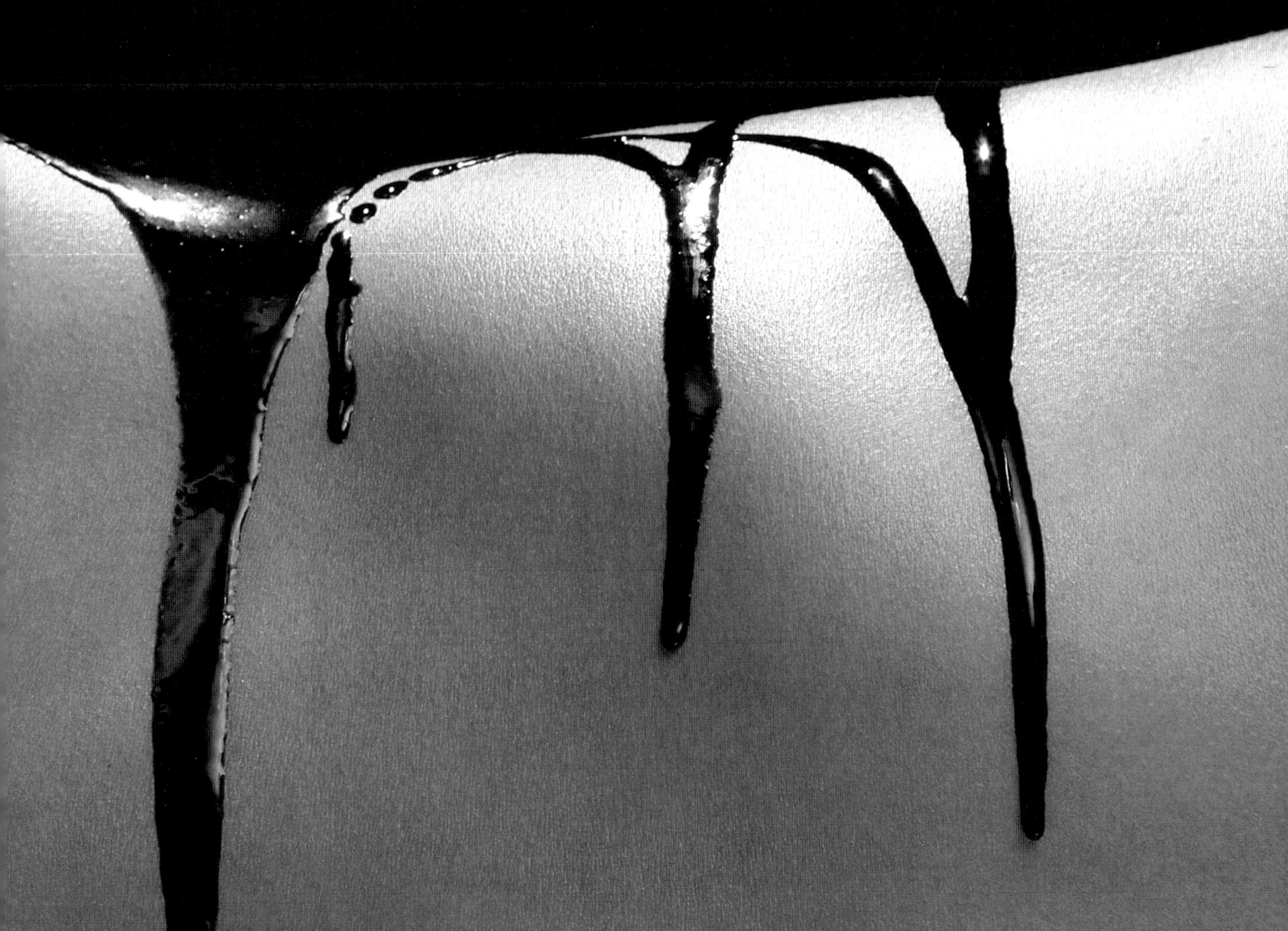

IMAGINE

I WILL ALWAYS REMEMBER MY FIRST experience at a five-star hotel. I had been traveling all day and I was exhausted and frazzled. But the minute I walked into the atrium lobby, I felt relief. I took the first deep breath I'd taken all day. My eyes fell upon the huge sculpture of beautiful fresh flowers in the center of the atrium. The perfume from the lilies lightly scented the entire lobby. The rugs and walls were rich and complex in both color and texture. The marble counters of the registration desk were cool and elegant. The lighting was indirect and flattering. As I caught my image in one of the large mirrors, I was startled to see that I looked far more refreshed than I felt. I walked to my room down halls lined with little flower vases placed just above eye level. Each held a single flower, stunningly lit by a tiny museum light from above.

Stepping into my room, I was greeted by a complimentary basket of perfectly ripened fruit, dark chocolate, and chilled champagne. I kicked off my shoes and felt my tired feet relax into the plush carpet. Soft music was playing on a surround-sound CD player by the bed.

As I tucked myself in, I sank into a deep, soft feather bed. I had a blissful night's sleep and I awoke to a breakfast of eggs, an English muffin, and a tiny, perfectly cooked filet mignon, all served on an immaculate tray with crystal glasses, fine china, and fresh flowers. Next, I had my choice of a shower, a bath, or a Jacuzzi in my own elegantly appointed marble bathroom.

At my every turn, I was surprised and delighted by some new taste, sound, vision, comfort, or scent. Each moment in this hotel revealed a new, previously undiscovered detail that gave me delight. There was no big bang of amazement over any one item—there did not need to be. My senses were in a constant, consistent, cumulative state of arousal. I was delighted to my core. It was just like great sex.

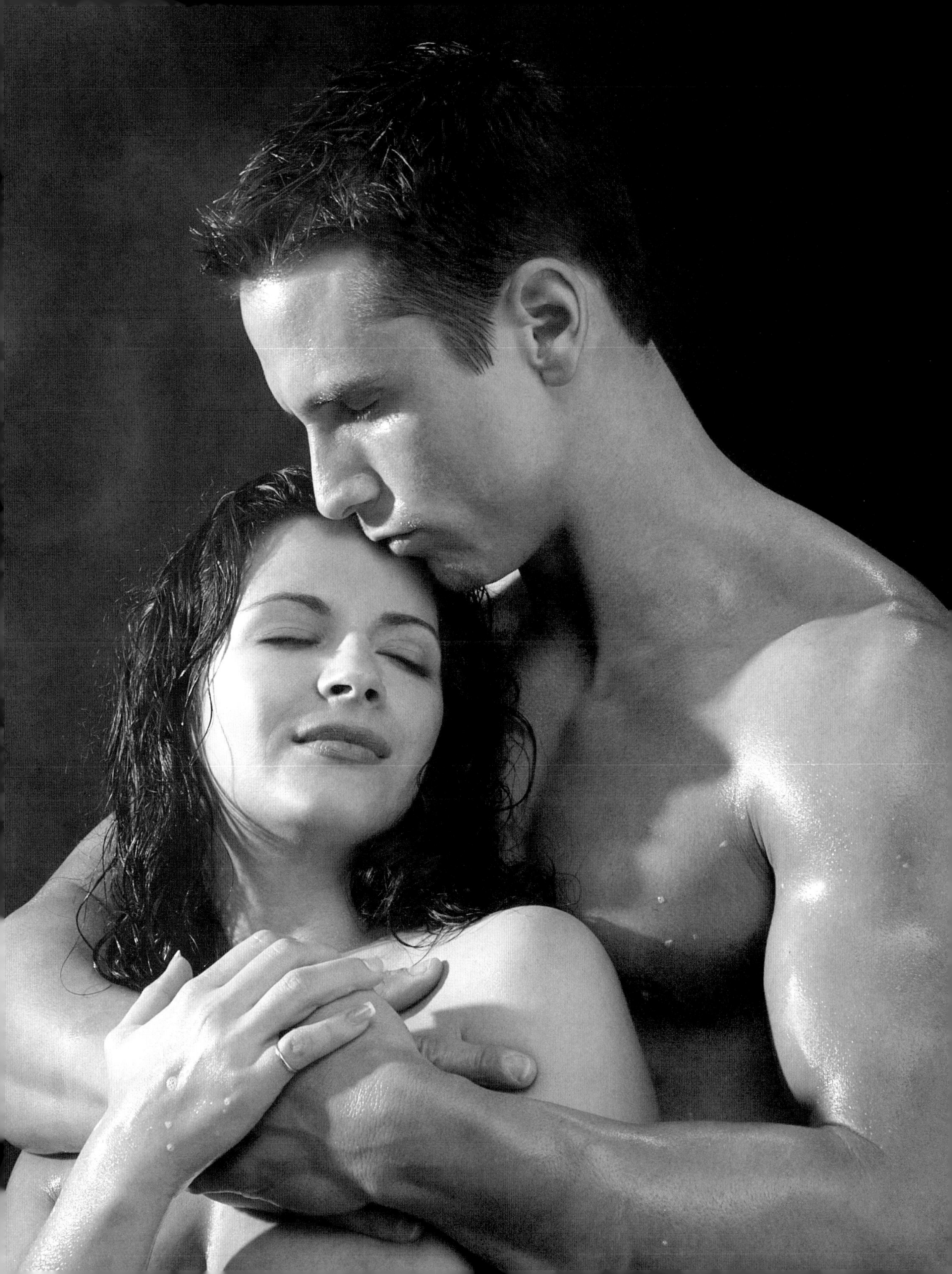

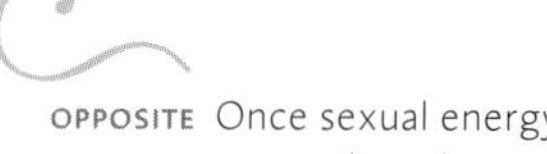

OPPOSITE Once sexual energy is in motion, you can use breath, touch, sound, and movement to build it and ride it like a wave.

Luxurious Loving, Luxurious Sex

There are lots of kinds of great sex. I am grateful to say that I have experienced a rich mélange of sex with many fascinating people. When I was younger, I favored intensity over intimacy. On some days, I still do. But over the course of both my personal and professional explorations of sex, I have found a style of sex that satisfies my passion for intensity as well as my desire for connection with both my partner and my inner self. It's a style of sex that I describe as luxurious.

Luxurious sex does not require a five-star hotel nor does it involve any great expenditures of money. Luxurious sex is specific to no special place or time period. Luxurious loving is a way of approaching love and sex that—like a five-star hotel—focuses on quality, not quantity. Luxurious loving is a process, not a goal. Return with me for a moment to my genuinely luxurious five-star hotel. The people who run this hotel make luxury a regular routine. The feather beds are fluffed daily. The flowers are replaced regularly. The chef consistently searches out new sources and menus for the freshest foods and finest wines. All these details must be attended to in order to achieve and maintain luxury. It's an ongoing process.

In a hotel where luxury is a goal instead of a process, things feel very different. At first glance, the hotel may look even more expensive and grand than the five-star hotel, but the beds aren't as soft, the air is not as fresh, the lighting is harsher and the imitation-brass doorknob may come off in your hand. You instinctively know that you are in faux luxury.

Sex is similar. Let's face it; most sex is good. There is no such thing as a bad orgasm. But we all know that some orgasms are prolonged, mind-blowing excursions into ecstasy and others are quiet, brief, and simply pleasant. There is certainly nothing wrong with a pleasant orgasm. But there is so much more to be enjoyed when orgasm is the inevitable next step in an already orgasmic *process*, not the winning goal at the end of a game.

Phases of Sexual Response

According to the legendary sex researchers Masters and Johnson, there are four phases of human sexual response: excitement, plateau, orgasm, and resolution. Biologically, here is what happens in each:

EXCITEMENT

The excitement phase can last anywhere from less than a minute to as long as several hours during which the clitoris, breasts, penis, and testes become engorged with blood. Heart rate and blood pressure increase. A man's penis becomes erect or partially erect and the testes elevate. In women, the clitoral shaft grows larger, the outer labia separate, and the inner labia enlarge, sometimes becoming darker in color. Women produce anywhere from a little to a lot of lubrication at this point.

PLATEAU

Contrary to the usual use of the word, plateau is not a leveling-off phase. It's a phase during which everything that happens during the excitement phase continues, becoming more and more intense. Sexual tension continues to grow as orgasm approaches. Both men and women will usually make involuntary sounds.

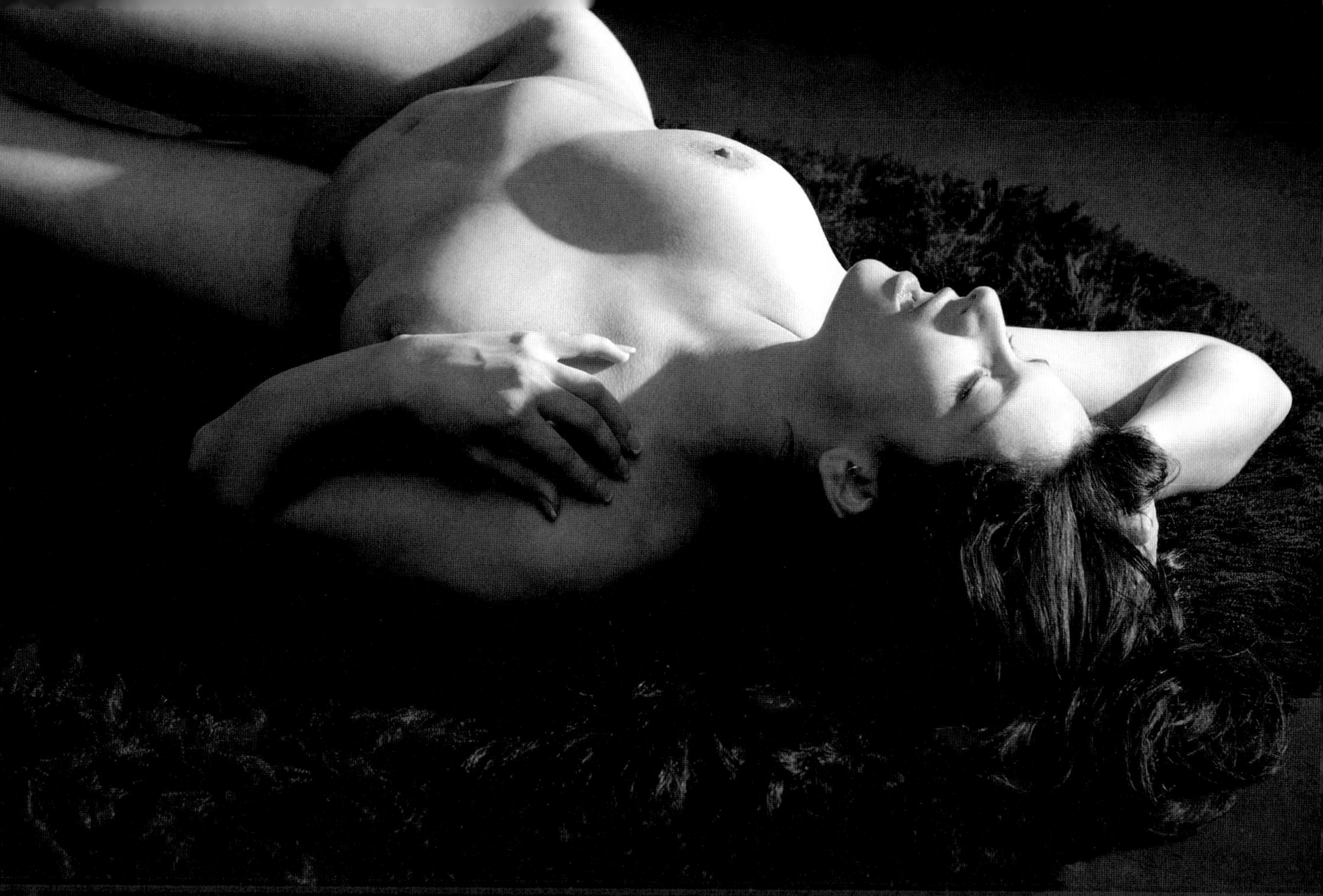

There is so much more to be enjoyed when orgasm is the inevitable next step in an already orgasmic process, not the winning goal at the end of a game.

ORGASM

According to Masters and Johnson, orgasm is the shortest phase of the cycle, typically lasting only several seconds. Men usually experience orgasm and ejaculation simultaneously, but ejaculation does not always occur at the time of orgasm. Prior to ejaculation, seminal fluids must gather in the ejaculatory ducts and upper urethra, producing a feeling that orgasm is inevitable. Semen is expelled from the penis at the time of ejaculation. When a woman orgasms, the uterus and pelvic floor contract in rhythmic waves of muscular movement.

RESOLUTION

If there is no additional stimulation, the resolution phase begins immediately after orgasm. In the resolution phase, the body returns to its original, nonexcited state. Some of the changes occur more rapidly than others.

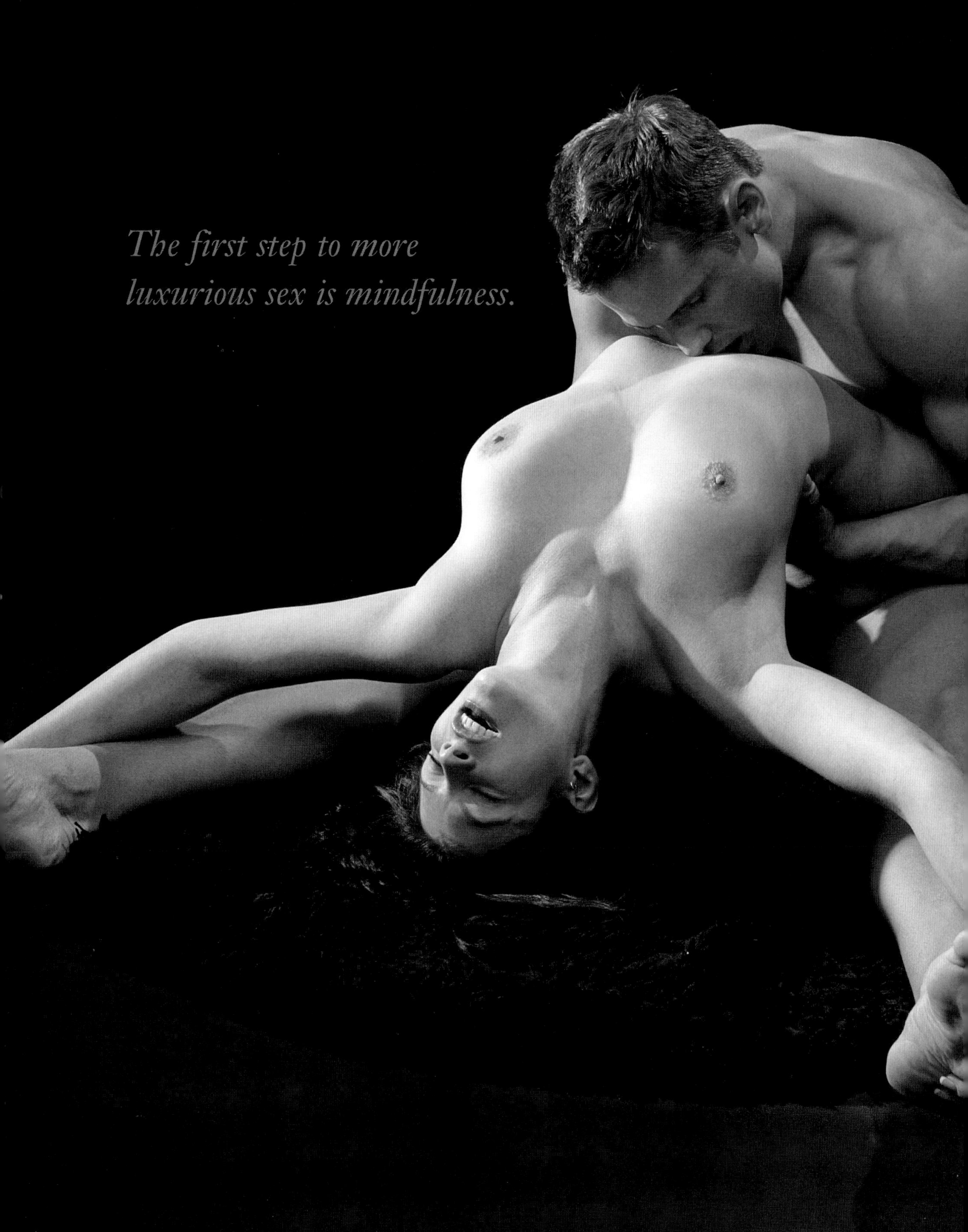
The first step to more luxurious sex is mindfulness.

Eastern Traditions

That's the biological, Western model of sexual response and it is accurate as far as it goes. Eastern cultures have approached sex quite differently. Tantra originated in India in the early centuries CE as a spiritual and social alternative to the popular religions of the day: Hinduism and Buddhism. Prior to Tantra, traditional beliefs held that enlightenment by which they meant a release from an endless cycle of death and rebirth—involved the renunciation of worldly pleasures. Each sect had its own opinions about exactly which pleasures should be the most conscientiously avoided and how best to avoid them.

SEX IS ENERGY

Tantra was quite different. It promised enlightenment in a single lifetime to those who cultivated, rather than avoided, pleasure, vision, and ecstasy. In the Tantric view of the creation of the world, Shiva, the god of pure consciousness, joins in sexual love with Shakti, the goddess of pure energy, giving birth to the world. Thus, Tantra views life, love, and sex as ongoing processes of creation on all levels at all times. In Tantra, sex is not an action. It is not one more thing humans *do*. Sex is an energy that exists on its own. All you have to do is notice it and it will start to move. Here's an example: Close your eyes. Put all your attention onto the index finger of your right hand. Breathe into the finger. Imagine a light shining inside this finger. Feel the blood pulsing in the finger. Do this for a couple of minutes. How does your finger feel? Bigger, more awake, and more alive, right? Energy follows thought. There is no difference between the energy you built in your finger and the energy you build in your genitals. Once sexual energy is in motion, you can use breath, touch, sound, and movement to build it and ride it like a wave.

Change Your Focus

Masters and Johnson's four-phase model of sexual response has unfortunately been used to reinforce a goal-oriented sexual style. In Tantra, when we focus not on the goal of orgasm but on excitement and arousal, we are, ironically, capable of longer orgasms, more intense orgasms, multiple orgasms, orgasms without ejaculation, and even new kinds of "energy" orgasms. The longer you stay in the excitement phase, the more hormones and endorphins are secreted by your glands, producing altered states of consciousness that can last for a long time, even after orgasm occurs. You can transcend thought and enter a world of pure sensation. In short, luxurious lovemaking can lead to a powerful and healthy natural high that can benefit your emotional, physical, and spiritual life.

SAVOR EACH MOMENT

The first step to more luxurious sex is mindfulness. All mindfulness means is attention to each successive moment: Here we are... here we are now... here we are now in this new moment. Each moment is sweet, savored. You don't have to go anywhere or do anything. Mindfulness is not multitasking. When we do more than one thing at a time, the adrenaline rush can certainly be energizing, but adrenaline is not ecstatic. It does not nourish us; it eventually burns us out. Mindfulness is its own reward. Let me demonstrate with a technique borrowed from Zen meditation.

If you can step outdoors for this exercise, so much the better. If you are indoors, position yourself so you are looking out a window, if possible. Stand with feet hip distance apart. Feel the ground through your feet. Keep your eyes open. Smile. Just be. Notice what you see and how you feel. Breathe. Now make a small move with your feet. Notice all the changes that

As in meditation, it is not difficult to practice mindfulness in sex. You are able to appreciate each present moment by keeping your attention focused on an intention.

have occurred in what you now observe, even though the move you made was very small. That's how mindfulness can magnify the smallest of actions.

CALM YOUR MIND WITH MEDITATION

The essence of luxurious loving—and luxurious living—is not in making huge changes. It is in noticing, appreciating, and maximizing the smallest of changes. The key to doing this is *slowing down*. This does not mean that you have to transform yourself from the busiest person in town to the slowest. It simply means that you have to learn to be able to slow down when you want to. One of the best ways to practice this is through meditation. There is nothing difficult, mysterious, or flaky about meditation. Meditation is simply the technique of calming the mind to access energy and insight. The nonanalytic, receptive state of meditation relieves pain and stress, boosts your immune system, and awakens your intuition. You can see results in as little as three minutes.

Try this three-minute heart meditation: Find a comfortable spot away from the distractions of phones, beepers, and people. Get comfortable. Snuggle into your favorite chair, get into a sensuous hot bath, or just sit in a favorite spot in your garden. Relax your body. Inhale slowly. Exhale slowly. Place your hand on your heart. Concentrate on something you love. It could be a person, a place, or a memory. (I like to imagine a puppy on my lap.) Breathe that feeling of love into your heart. Keep your attention focused on your breath and your heart. If outside thoughts come up, don't engage them, just notice them and let them float away. Notice any sensations that happen in your heart center. You might feel warmth, coolness, vibrations, tingling, expansion, security, compassion, or bliss. Let the feeling expand and flow out through your body. Don't worry if you don't feel anything at first. The point is not to feel anything specific but to just be still and authentic. When you can allow your body to be still and your mind to be quiet, your senses open. Mind chatter is like a white-noise machine—it can keep you from experiencing all manner of exquisite sensations, especially in lovemaking.

Meditation teaches mindfulness. Mindfulness produces more mindfulness, which, in sex, leads to more bliss. As in meditation, it is not difficult to practice mindfulness in sex. You are able to appreciate each present moment by keeping your *attention* focused on an *inten-*

OPPOSITE Treat your lover with kindness, reverence, and devotion both in and out of the bedroom.

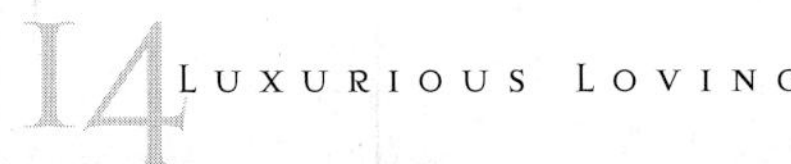

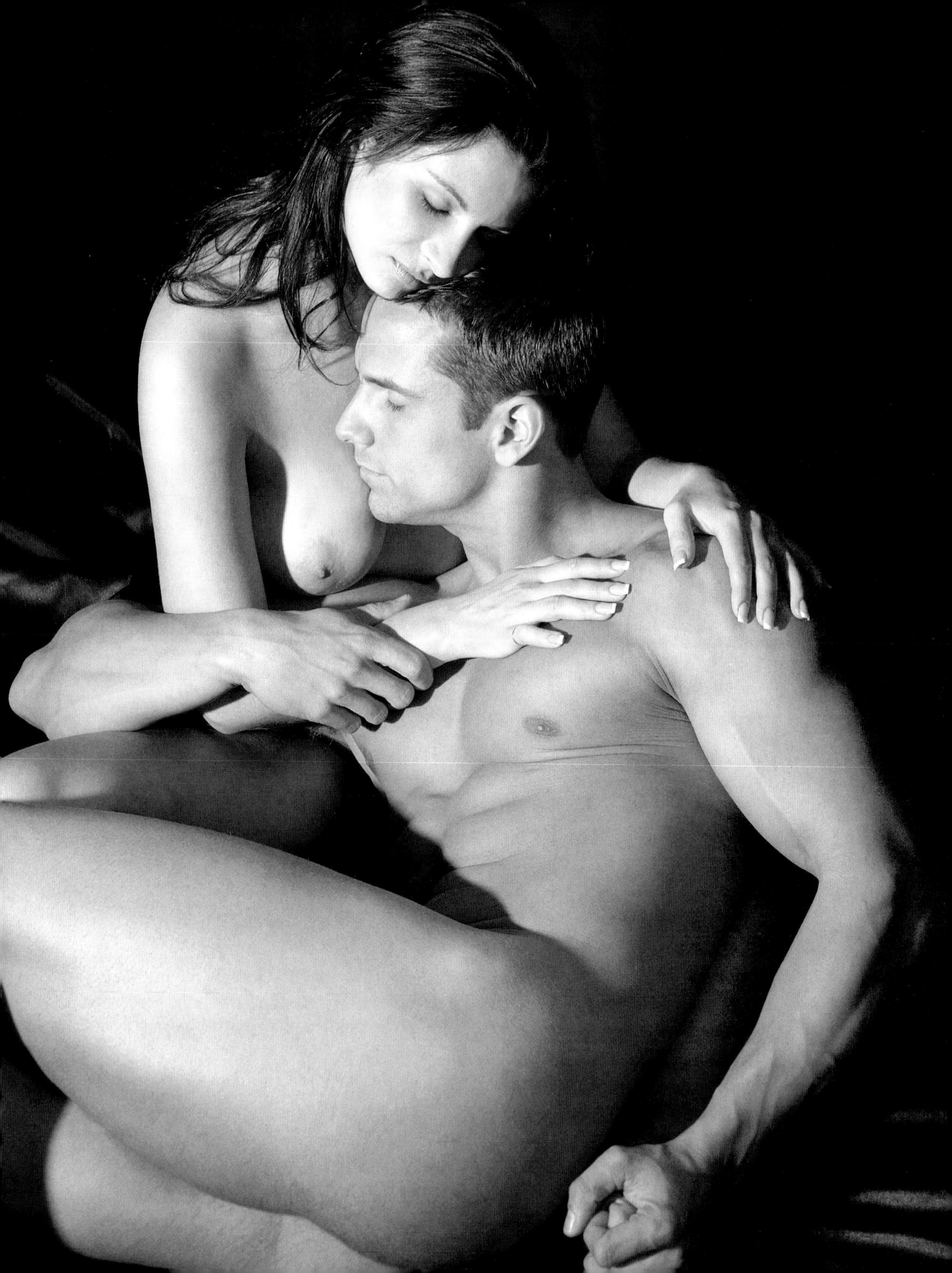

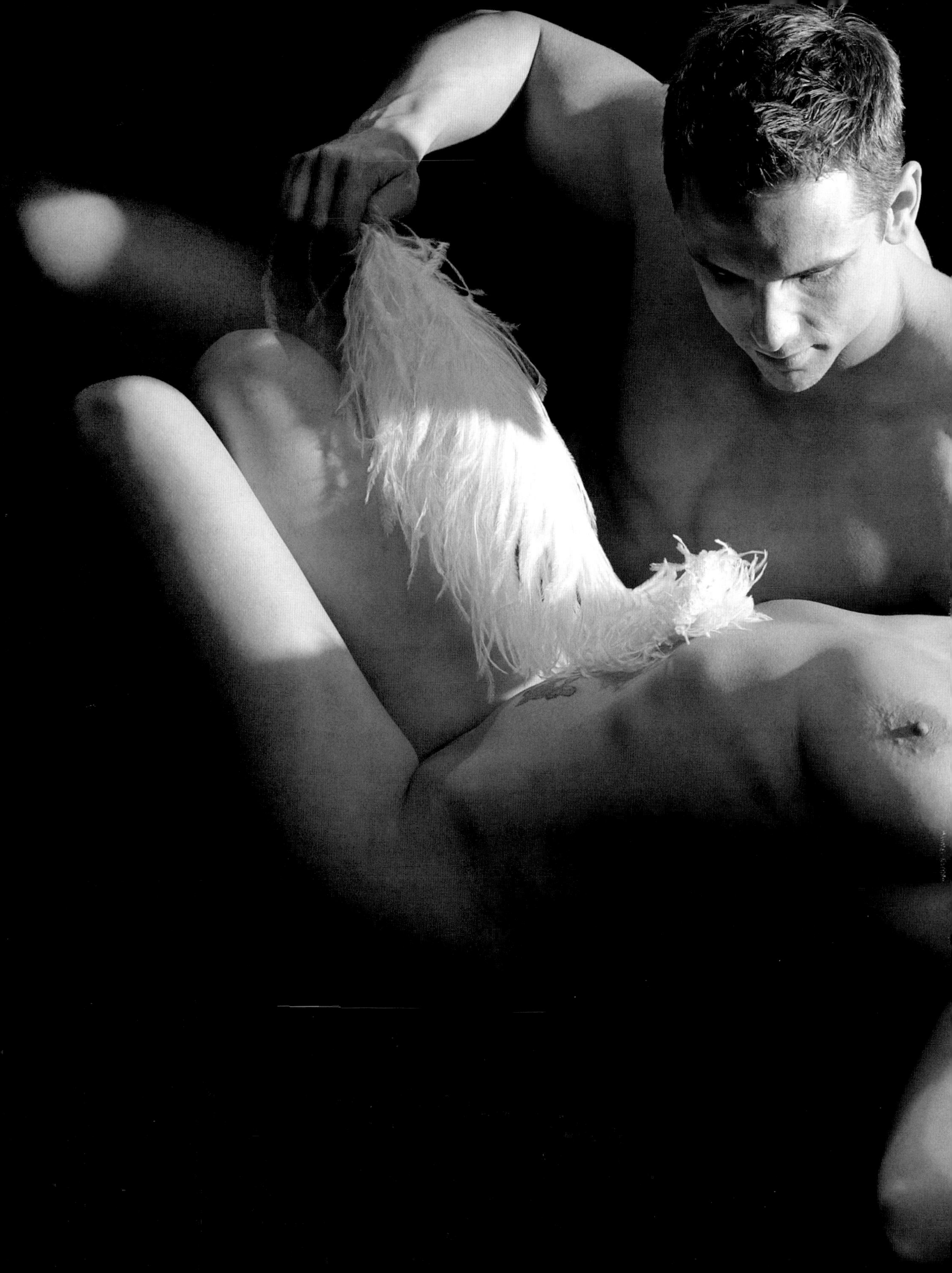

When you slow down and put your attention where your intention is, you will be able to build and circulate more sexual energy than you ever imagined.

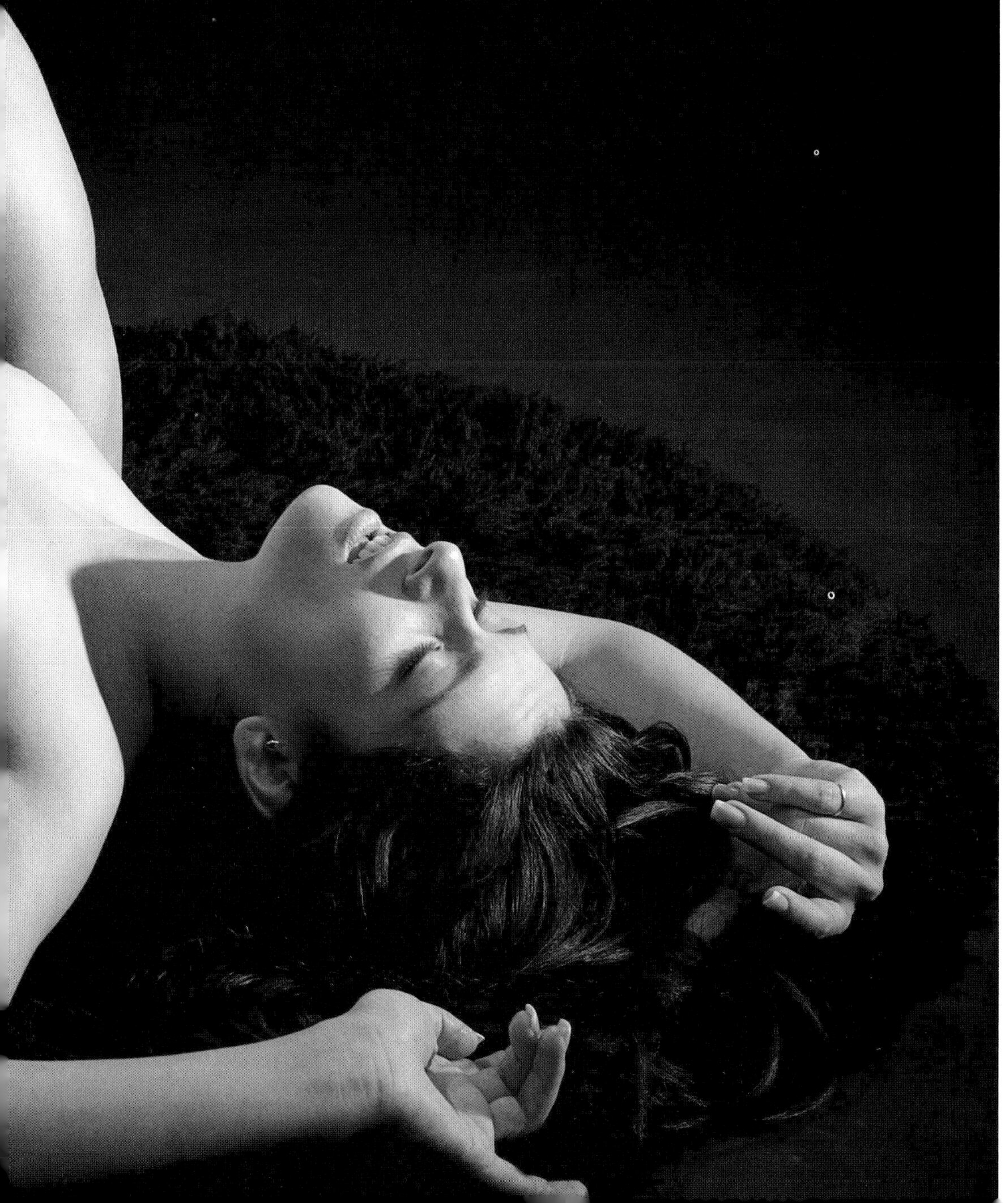

tion. For example, your intention may be to give your partner pleasure with your hands in a sensuous massage. In this case you would keep your attention on your hands and on the response your lover's body gives you as you caress her. If your intention is to enjoy the exquisite touch of your lover's tongue as he gives you oral sex, you might send each breath you take into your genitals to help you keep your attention on your clitoris. If your intention is to build a massive wave of sexual energy with your lover and ride it for as long as you can, your attention will be focused on the techniques that build that energy. When you slow down and put your attention where your intention is, you will be able to build and circulate more sexual energy than you ever imagined.

Come to Your Senses

Attentiveness to intention also helps us break the mindless, hurried sexual habits we have all accumulated over time. Most of these habits relate to goals and expectations, such as that a kiss will lead to sex or that orgasm is the necessary climax of every sexual encounter. When we focus on building extended states of intense arousal, there are no goals. Climax becomes a process. Emphasizing the excitement phase of lovemaking is like climbing a staircase to heaven. On each floor you experience a new level of pleasure that nourishes you, transforms you, and prepares you for the next level. When the excitement phase is prolonged, the other stages of sex—plateau, orgasm, and resolution—are more profound and occur automatically. The orgasm produced in this way is more intense and the resolution phase is longer and deeper. You can try a version of this right now.

Devote a week to "coming to your senses." Spend a week without intercourse or orgasm as you use the techniques in this book to open up all your senses. Devote some time each day to building erotic energy with your lover by diving into the delicious depths of breath, smell, taste, touch, movement, sight, and sound. At the end of the week, allow your erotic explorations to climax with orgasm and afterglow.

Mindfulness is applicable not only to the body. It is also applicable to relationships. How do you and your lover treat each other when you are not in bed? Are you kind to each other—*truly* kind? Or are the two of you prone to misunderstandings and hurt feelings? Make a vow to treat each other with more day-to-day reverence and kindness. Think back to when the two of you had just fallen in love. Your lover was a god or a goddess in your eyes. You could not do enough for him or her and every word he or she spoke was fascinating. You went out of your way to show your beloved every possible courtesy and affection. The ardent feelings that produce this loving, considerate behavior are produced by physical changes in brain chemistry, and, unfortunately, this phase of passionate sexual and emotional intensity rarely lasts longer than eighteen to twenty-four months. However, lovemaking that focuses on mindful awareness, slowing down, and breathing consciously can produce changes in brain chemistry that can do much to bring back that state. We are all highly suggestible when we are highly aroused—the mind becomes like a sponge. When you communicate kindly and gently and with an attitude of devotion, loyalty, equality, and kindness, intimacy and trust deepen. Words spoken during lovemaking that could be interpreted as critical, demeaning, or thoughtless can sow the seeds of future problems in your relationship. When you develop a mindful, considerate relationship with your lover outside the bedroom, you make love with mindfulness, trust, and closeness already in place.

When you achieve your sexual goals, what will the rest of your life look like? What will your sexual transformation do for your relationships, your career, your playtime?

IMAGINE THE POSSIBILITIES

It's often said that the most important sex organ is the brain. This is a biological fact. Erotic energy may begin in your genitals, but it's the mind that takes over from there. The mind can say yes or no to any particular expression of erotic energy. Most of what works or doesn't work in your sex life and in your life in general is based on a belief or a limitation you hold in your mind.

What is your sex life like now?
What would make it better?

Once you have the answer to both of those questions, you can use your imagination to expand the answer to the second question. For example, if you know you're capable of so much more sexually and you'd like to be able to find out what that is, imagine what that *might* look like. There is no right or wrong answer and you can always change your mind. So go wild. Imagine this new expanded sex life. What would great sex feel like, taste like, smell like, and sound like? What are the qualities of a great sex life for you? No matter how small or how grand your sexual ambition, imagine it. Keep focused on yourself, rather than on a real or imagined partner. You are creating your *own* expanded, delicious, exquisite, and totally hot new sex life—not your partner's. Your partner may make an appearance in your imaginings, but he or she is not the key to your sex life. *You* are. What you believe is possible for you *is* possible for you.

Now take your imaginings a step further. When you achieve your sexual goals, what will the rest of your life look like? What will your sexual transformation do for your relationships, your career, your playtime? Imagine the power and pleasure of your new sex life washing over your entire life and making every moment luxurious, powerful, and precious.

Let's start climbing the stairway to heaven that is luxurious loving. You can start anywhere in this book and move through the chapters in any order. At each step along the path your imagination will help take you to the next level. All is possible.

Breathe

BREATHE

2

Take a *deep* breath. Send your breath deep down until you can feel it tickle your genitals from the inside.

Exhale slowly.

Take a *full* breath. Let your breath expand your rib cage. Let your belly fill with air. Let breath fill the spaces under your shoulder blades.

Exhale slowly.

Now take a *deep, full* breath. Take in as much air as you can and let it expand you laterally and vertically.

Exhale with a big sound.

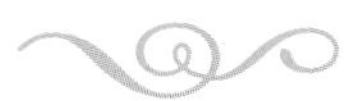

IT MAY BE HARD TO BELIEVE, BUT YOU just took the single most important step you may ever take toward great sex. Breath is your greatest source of energy and aliveness. It can produce so much pleasure, it will amaze you. Once you become familiar with moving erotic energy around with and on your breath, you'll find all your erotic encounters to be much more fulfilling. Your orgasms will be longer and deeper. You will share a more authentically intimate connection with your partner. You'll even find yourself using breath techniques in nonerotic situations to bring erotic energy to more and more areas of your life.

Most of us breathe just enough to stay alive but not enough to really feel our aliveness. Think of a physical activity you really enjoy. It might be skiing or running, dancing or walking on the beach. If you're not fond of physical activity, think of someone on television who has just completed a race or any act of physical endurance. What is the most obvious physical response occurring in the bodies of those who have just participated in a physical

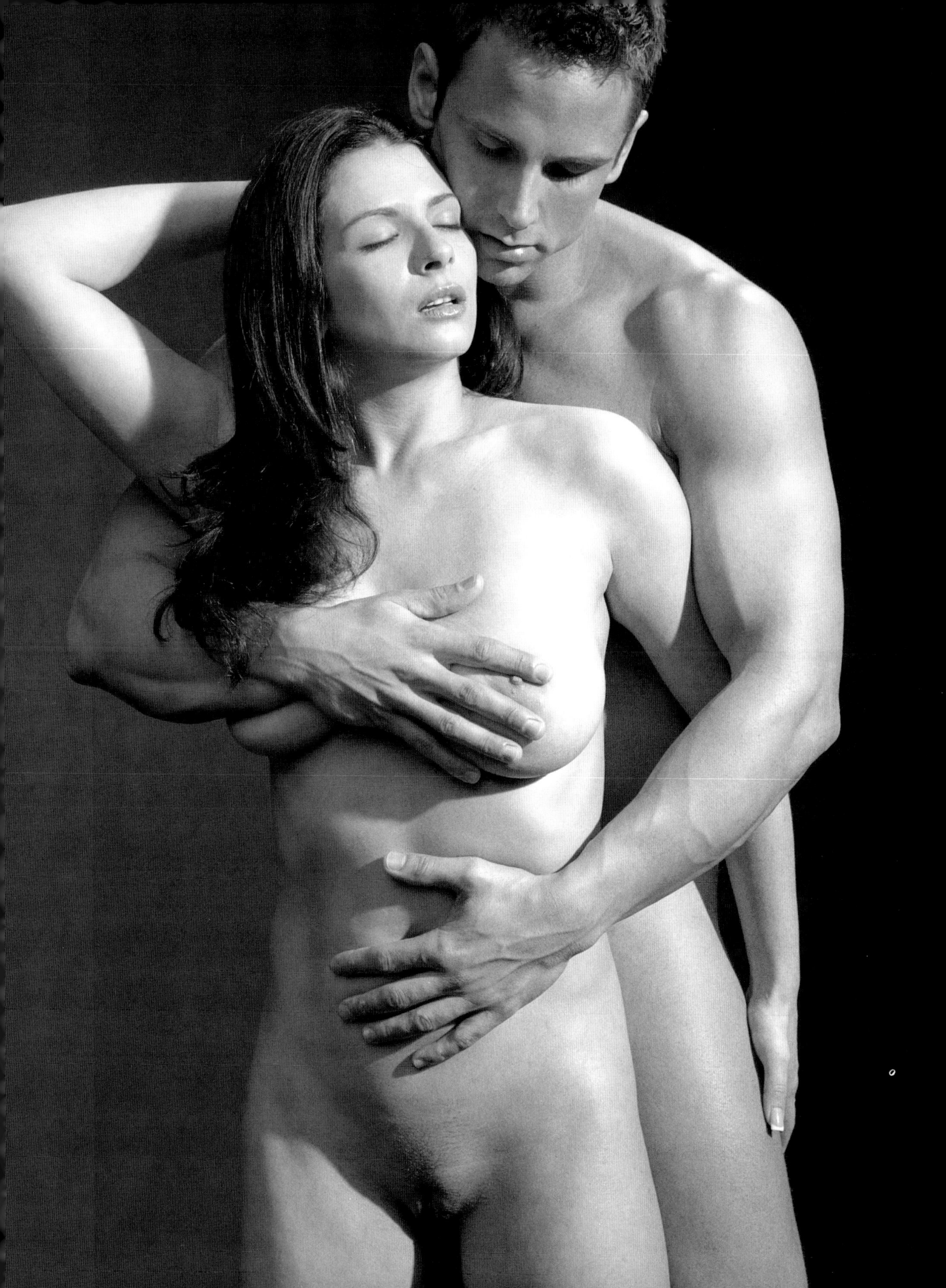

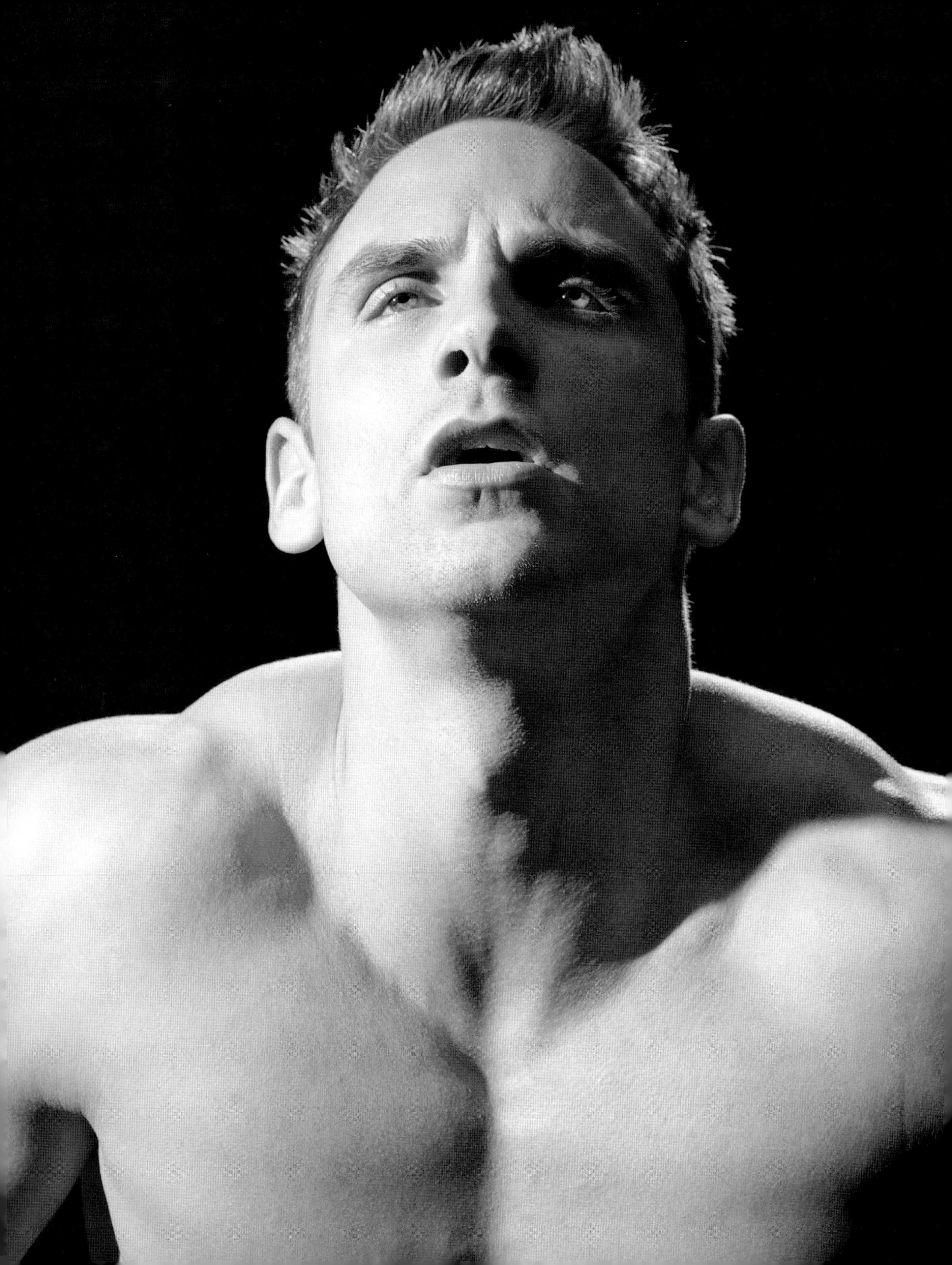

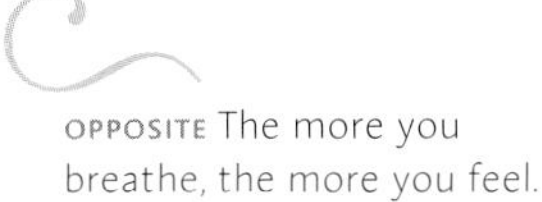

OPPOSITE The more you breathe, the more you feel.

activity they enjoy? They are taking *big deep breaths.* They may be breathing so hard that they can barely talk. They may seem completely drained, but they don't care. There is an aura of extra aliveness around them. They are enjoying a peak experience—the combination of physical activity and conscious breathing has produced euphoria. The same thing happens in sex. Intense physical activity plus conscious breathing equals euphoria. Of course we get an enormous amount of pleasure from our genitals and most of us have had orgasms while clenching, bearing down, and holding our breath. But the orgasms that result from those compressed quickies are short and localized to the genital area. When you want to stay in the excitement phase of lovemaking for as long as possible and enjoy extended orgasmic states, it is your breath, not your genitals, that will hold you in the totality of ever-increasing sensation.

Conscious Breathing

Just as in sports or dancing or yoga, it is not only the way you breathe that is important. It is also essential that you *keep breathing consistently* throughout the game or dance or class. It's the same in sex. We call this conscious—or mindful—breathing. That means that you stay aware of your breathing. You put your *attention* where your *intention* is. For example, imagine that your lover is giving you exquisite oral sex. This lover seems psychic. Everyplace he puts his lips and tongue is exactly right and leads to increasingly exquisite pleasure. All you need to do is to move ever so slightly so that your genitals meet his mouth in one perfect combination after the other. This dance of your subtle movement and your lover's mouth seems to go on endlessly until it finally builds into a rocketlike orgasm that picks you up and hurls you off the earth and into the cosmos. You are being mindful of moving your clitoris or penis into exactly the right, ever-changing position. Your intention is to receive maximum pleasure. Your attention is on the precise spot on your genitals that feels better than any other spot. You are putting your attention where your intention is. It's a very effective—and pleasurable—use of mindfulness/consciousness. To prolong passion and increase sensation in your practice of luxurious loving, you'll want to apply that same mindfulness to your breath. It will take a little practice, but the rewards will be surprisingly greater than the results of the mindfulness you have been giving to your genitals.

There are three things you need to know about breath and sex:

1. Changing the way you breathe changes the way you feel.
2. Sexual energy travels on the breath.
3. The more you breathe, the more you feel.

HEART BREATH

Here is a simple mindful breath technique called the Heart Breath that will help you understand the connection between breath and pleasure:

Yawn. Try to yawn the biggest, fullest, most rewarding yawn you can. (If you don't actually get a yawn out of this, that's okay. A huge big fake yawn is nearly as effective.) Do you feel how the yawn opens the back of your throat and stretches out your whole mouth and face? That's the feeling of openness you want when you do the Heart Breath.

Now let your mouth fall open slightly. Relax your jaw and face, open the back of your throat, and breathe in through your mouth, gently but fully. Exhale. Don't push the breath out; just let it fall out of your body with a gentle little sigh, *ahhh*. Take in as much air as you can—as effortlessly as you can—then let it go.

Keep on breathing just like that.

Erotically speaking, this simple breath can take you almost anywhere you want to go. You can speed it up or slow it way down. You can take in a lot of air with a minimum of effort and tension. Simple as this breath is, you will need to practice it to enjoy its power and pleasures. Start with ten minutes of constant, conscious breathing. Remember, your intention is to breathe the Heart Breath for ten minutes. Therefore, you'll need to put your attention on your breath. Sit comfortably and keep your eyes open. Gently focus them on a point across the room. When you are sitting upright with your eyes open, you won't nod off or space out. You can set a timer, so you don't have to keep track of the time. When your time is up, take three deeper breaths and then breathe normally. Notice how you feel.

In what ways do you feel different from how you felt before breathing the Heart Breath? You may feel peaceful, relaxed, light-headed, tingly (especially in your hands or face), or even a little stoned. That's the physical reality of conscious breathing. It produces a change in consciousness. Breath is a conscious sexual technique that we can use at any time to control and intensify our pleasure. We can create an unlimited range of sexual possibilities that we never would have discovered if we simply let our breathing be the haphazard result of sexual activity.

Move Energy All Through Your Body

Now let's experiment with using your breath to move sexual energy throughout your body. Lie back in a comfortable position. Place one hand on your genitals and your other hand on your heart. Begin to masturbate (you can use a vibrator if you'd like). Breathe. Imagine that each time you inhale, your sexual energy travels up from your genitals to your heart. Keep your focus on both your breathing and the sensation of pleasure in your genitals. Just before you are about to orgasm, stop masturbating and breathe all that orgasmic feeling up into your heart. Keep breathing and let that orgasm sensation expand in your heart until it fills your entire chest. Now begin to masturbate again. Continue the breath and the genital-to-heart visualization. Once again, stop masturbating just before orgasm, and again breathe that orgasm into your heart. This time let the sensation travel out from your heart, down your arms into your hands. At this point you may—or may not—experience involuntary muscle twitches called *kriyas*. Kriyas happen when tension in the body releases. Imagine that your body is a coiled garden hose. When you turn on the water (sexual energy), the hose tends to twitch around until the water pressure causes it to straighten out enough for the water to flow easily. Kriyas can be very pleasurable. If you breathe into them, they can multiply and turn into little energy orgasms that dance around your body.

For a third time, begin to masturbate. Reestablish your mindful practice of the Heart Breath. Breathe in through your mouth, gently but fully. When you exhale, let your breath fall out with a gentle sound. This time, let yourself orgasm genitally at the same time you also breathe the orgasm into your heart. Then simply relax. Don't try to make anything happen. Just be.

How was this erotic meditation different from your usual self-loving? What effect did the mindful use of breath have on your orgasm? Were you able to feel the sexual energy moving through your body? Were your heartgasms as intense or nearly as intense as your genital orgasm? Was your genital orgasm longer or deeper than usual? It may have taken you longer to reach orgasm while you werebreathing mindfully. This is good! It means that your breath was moving your sexual energy around your body. When we masturbate by

When we breathe fully and consciously, it's like filling a five-gallon jug instead of a coffee cup. It takes longer, but the payoff is a bigger, deeper, longer orgasm and a more delicious afterglow.

holding our breath and bearing down (the classic quickie), we limit our sexual energy to the area around our genitals. When we breathe fully and consciously, it's like filling a five-gallon jug instead of a coffee cup. It takes longer, but the payoff is a bigger, deeper, longer orgasm and a more delicious afterglow. The more you breathe, the more you feel and the more you will realize that the only limits to pleasure and sensation in your body are the limits of your imagination. When you open yourself up to more possibilities of pleasure, you find them and then you can imagine even more possibilities. The process is infinite. As you and your partner commit to your exploration of the excitement phase of lovemaking, you enter the universe of unlimited pleasure.

ENERGY ORGASMS

Here's a new possibility for you to consider: You can orgasm nongenitally simply by breathing. These orgasms are called *energy orgasms*. Energy orgasms feel a bit different from genital orgasms (though you could possibly have a genital orgasm and an energy orgasm at the same time). Energy orgasms are full-body orgasmic experiences. Instead of starting in your genitals, it feels as if the orgasmic energy starts in the very center of your being, then flows out to the limits of your body and beyond. You may feel free from boundaries, as though you can't tell where "you" end and "everything else" begins. You may even inhabit an alternative universe where everything is beautiful, quiet, and peacefully interconnected. Your orgasm may seem to be happening everywhere and nowhere, and it can go on and on and on. After an energy orgasm, you may feel energized or you may feel peaceful and blissed out. Energy-orgasm techniques vary, but practicing any energy-orgasm technique will help you expand your concept of sex, pleasure, and orgasm. One very simple yet very powerful technique is the Clench and Hold.

Clench and Hold Lie comfortably on your back on the floor. Relax your jaw. Yawn. Keep the back of your throat open. Breathe using the Heart Breath. Take in as much air as you can with the least possible effort. Keep your eyes open, focused on a point somewhere on the ceiling, because you want to stay aware of your breath and not nod off. If you want, you can gently rock your hips as you breathe. Allow all of this to be erotic. Just let it feel good. Remember to stay mindful of your breath. Set a timer and breathe for ten minutes, twenty, thirty, or more! The more you breathe, the more you'll charge your body with energy. When your timer goes off, you're ready to do the Clench and Hold. Take three deep full breaths. Release the first two breaths with sighs or sounds. On the third breath, hold it in, squeeze your buttocks together and tighten your lower abdomen as hard as you can. When you clench the lower abdomen, you'll usually find that the rest of your body wants to clench as well. That's just fine. You can enhance the clench by scrunching up your face and pressing down into the floor with your hands and shoulders, head and buttocks, legs and feet.

Keep clenching for about fifteen seconds, then let go. Let go completely. Just be. Don't try to make anything happen. Surrender. Some people have a great catharsis, some see visions or feel new sensations, some find a deep sense of inner peace. Each of these experiences is both valuable and useful. *Bigger is not better.* The Clench and Hold is an exercise in authenticity—in trusting the inner, nonconscious parts of your being. When you completely let go, you allow yourself to be guided by your inner wisdom toward an original and deep experience. Some people experience gigglegasms. Others have deep crygasms or intense angergasms. Still others have quiet blissgasms. When we stop thinking of orgasm as a purely genital experience, we open ourselves up to an entire universe of expanded orgasmic possibilities that I think of as training for sexual compassion. Compassion literally means "to feel together." When we allow ourselves to fully feel, express, and be, we gain the strength and ability to allow full sexual expression for both ourselves and our lovers.

Breathing Together

Thus far we have practiced erotic breath work as a solo technique. What happens when you are with a partner? How can you focus on both your partner and your breathing at the same time? Simple: You breathe together. Try it. Stand, sit, or lie beside or behind your partner. Simply match your breath to his. Stay focused on breathing at the same speed, rhythm, and depth with him. Keep your eyes open so as not to trance out or allow your mind to wander. After five or ten minutes, take a deep breath together and share with your partner how you are feeling. Are you relaxed? Agitated? Worried? Excited? Turned on? Ask your partner how he is feeling. You may very well find that you have "read" his mood. When we breathe with someone we are more able to feel what he is feeling. This is extremely useful in sex. This is not to say that you are expected to read your lover's mind! We all know what thorny brambles we can get tangled in when we skip blindly down that path. However, breath is a form of nonverbal connection that we can use to both listen and speak to our partner.

Breath is especially handy when one or the other of you would like to change your mood to something more pleasurable and words just won't do the trick. Let's say you come home from work early. You've had a great day. You are in a terrific mood that has just been improved by the fact that you have a couple of extra hours all by yourself to have a bath and read your new book. Your partner comes home three hours later, frazzled and drained. Her day has been a complete horror. She is angry and frustrated, but she is open to being comforted. After you have given her a little time to calm down and get comfortable, sit behind her on the floor or on the bed. At first she may be too tense to want to lean back against you and relax. Breathe with her for a minute. This will give you a sense of what she is feeling. Now change your breath to a calmer, fuller one. Make the change obvious. Exaggerate a little so she can more easily pick up the new rhythm. After she has matched her breath to yours, slow and deepen your breath even more. Make it easy for her to follow.

OPPOSITE The Breath Kiss is a delicious way to enjoy mindful breathing with a partner.

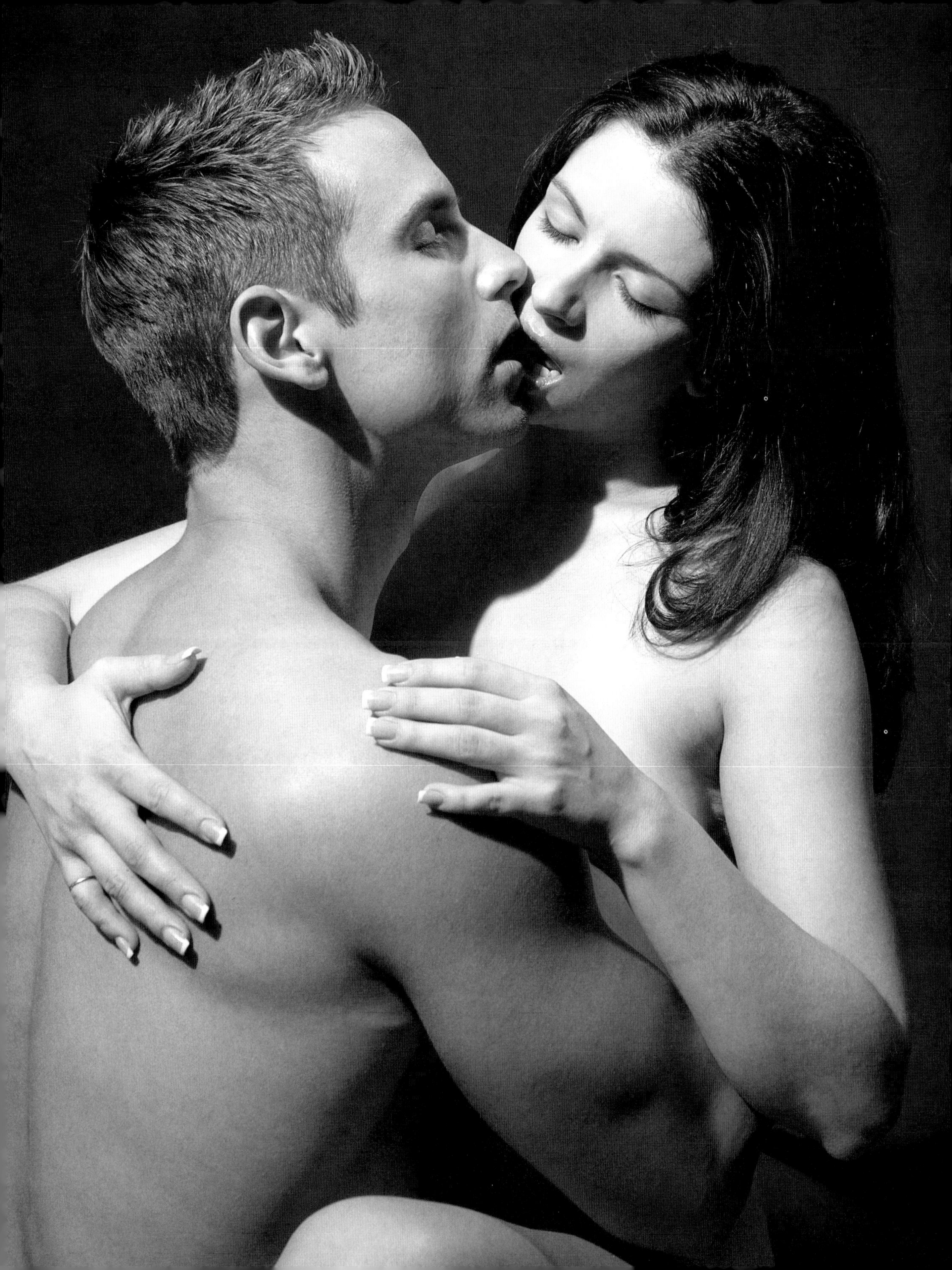

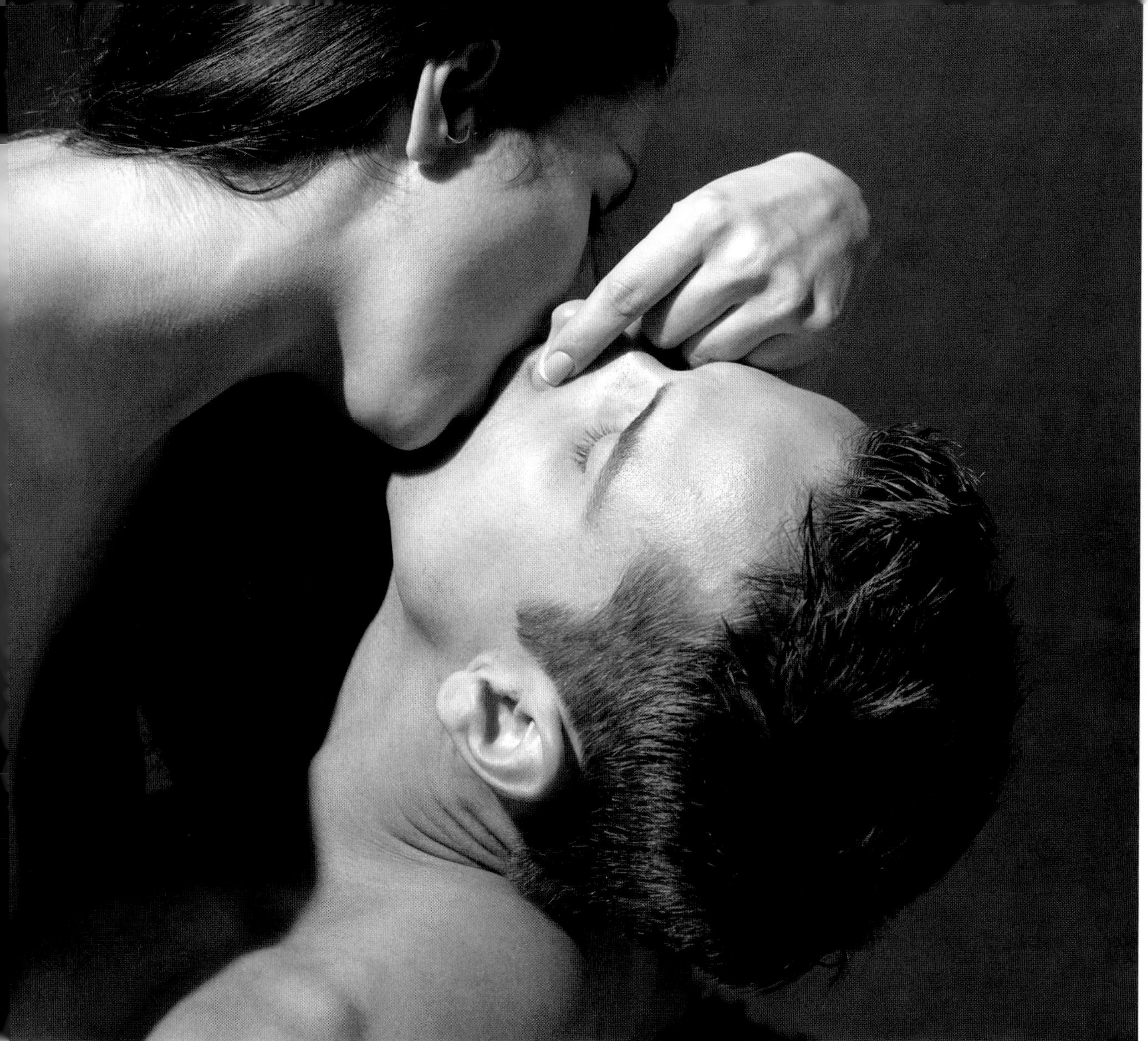

Your shared goal is a relaxed but alive state of being. Relaxation is an open, aware, awake state of being. You have a sense of energy flowing through you. Relaxation is not numb or floppy. When you are completely inert, movement of any kind is inhibited—there is no energy flowing. This state resembles tension more than it does relaxation.

MOUTH BREATHING

You can use your breath to relax your body or to charge it. Mouth breathing is a charging mechanism. We breathe through the mouth when we need or want more oxygen—for pleasure as well as survival. Although it is considered linked to our response to stress, breathing through our mouths can be more than the primitive human fight-or-flight response. Have you ever seen people in the throes of passion breathing through their noses with their mouths closed? Of course not. Mouth

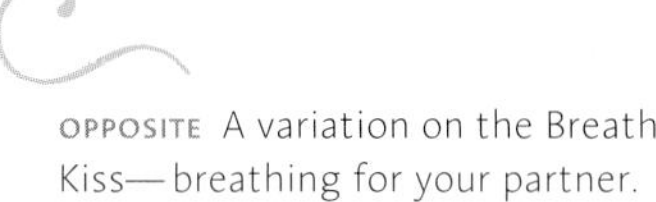

OPPOSITE A variation on the Breath Kiss—breathing for your partner.

breathing charges the body. When you learned the Heart Breath, you breathed in and out through your mouth because you wanted to increase your sexual energy and move it throughout your body.

NOSE BREATHING

When you breathe through your nose, air goes to the lower lobes of your lungs and stimulates the vagus nerve, part of the parasympathetic nervous system: the body's rest-and-restore system. The parasympathetic nervous system lowers heart rate and blood pressure, and sets in motion other calming measures to allow the body to rest, recover, and gain new energy. You can breathe through your nose to calm yourself in any number of situations: being stopped by a police officer, delaying ejaculation, and prolonging pleasure, to name a few.

Let's get back to your frazzled partner. After you have helped her relax with some minutes of slow and easy nose breathing, you can start a more energizing breath, breathing easily through your mouth and exhaling with a sigh. Keep in mind that you are not trying to manipulate your partner into sex. You are simply assisting her to find a state of relaxed aliveness. She always has the option of breathing along with you or breathing at her own rate. Once she is relaxed, she may have a good cry or a good scream, or she just may want you to screw her brainless. All are good. When we love luxuriously, our sole goal is to stay in the present moment, where all things are possible.

Practice breathing during sexual activities in which you normally breathe very little. For example, it can be hard to remember to breathe when you are lip-locked in an endless kiss.

BREATH KISS

The Breath Kiss is an incredibly pleasurable way to practice mindful breathing during partner sex. Join your lover in an open-mouthed kiss. As you breathe in, your lover breathes out, into your mouth. As you breathe out, he breathes in. Although you will actually be taking some air in through your nose, it will feel as if your partner is breathing for you. It may take a few moments for you to sync up the in and out breaths. Stay with it. Kiss for many minutes. Get lost in the kiss and the breath. This is a powerful technique. You may experience altered consciousness or enter a trancelike state. Enjoy it!

If you want to leap into the deep end of the intimacy and trust pool, try this variation of the Breath Kiss. Hold your partner's nose. Place your mouth over his and breathe for him. This is not a joke. You are really breathing for your partner. This is a trust exercise of the highest order. Your commitment must be total. And as with anything you commit yourself to completely, the rewards are potentially astounding. Your partner may feel a complete surrender, not only to you but to life and god. You may both experience new dimensions of compassion, tenderness, and love.

The mindful use of breath will transform your lovemaking. It may take a while before you ease into a completely new, breath-filled sex life. That's fine. There is no rush. Every time you practice, you will expand and enhance your lovemaking. Start slowly. Think ahead and plan how you can add breath to your favorite erotic activities. Make up sexy games that focus on breathing. When you are making love, remind your lover to breathe and ask him to do the same for you. Remember, everything feels better with breath.

3 SNIFF

HUMANS HAVE LONG USED THE luxury of scent to attract and seduce a mate. When Cleopatra sailed to meet Mark Anthony, the sails of her barge were scented to announce her arrival. In 800 BCE, the Queen of Sheba took fragrance to seduce Solomon. In ancient Rome, brides and grooms wore crowns of roses and their marriage beds were scented with rose petals. The mindful use of scent has always had the magical effect of unplugging our conscious mind and connecting us with our unconscious memories. It can lay the psychic and physical groundwork for intense arousal.

The sense of smell is our most ancient, primordial sense. The olfactory nerve travels straight to the most primitive part of the brain—the limbic system—which governs memory and emotions, bypassing the cerebral cortex—the conscious "thinking" part of the brain. That is why what we smell can stimulate our most primal sexual urges. In addition, our olfactory system puts us in direct physical contact with our surroundings. The beginning of the olfactory nerve sits at the top of the nasal cavity and is the only part of the human nervous system that is directly exposed to the environment. Yoga doctrines hold that breathing through the nose extracts the *prana* (also known as chi, or life-force energy) from the air. In Eastern sexual traditions, the nose is considered the psychic genitalia, providing pleasure to the mental and spiritual bodies the way our genitals provide pleasure to our physical bodies.

Our sense of smell is directly linked to our sexuality in physical ways as well. The nose is lined with an erectile tissue similar to that of our nipples and genitals. When we are exposed to particular scents that please us, the genital center is awakened. Scent is so integrated with our sexuality that without our sense of smell, our libido can decline sharply. Masters and Johnson noted that 25 percent of people with smell disorders lose interest in sex. Conversely, the mindful use of scent can dramatically enhance passion.

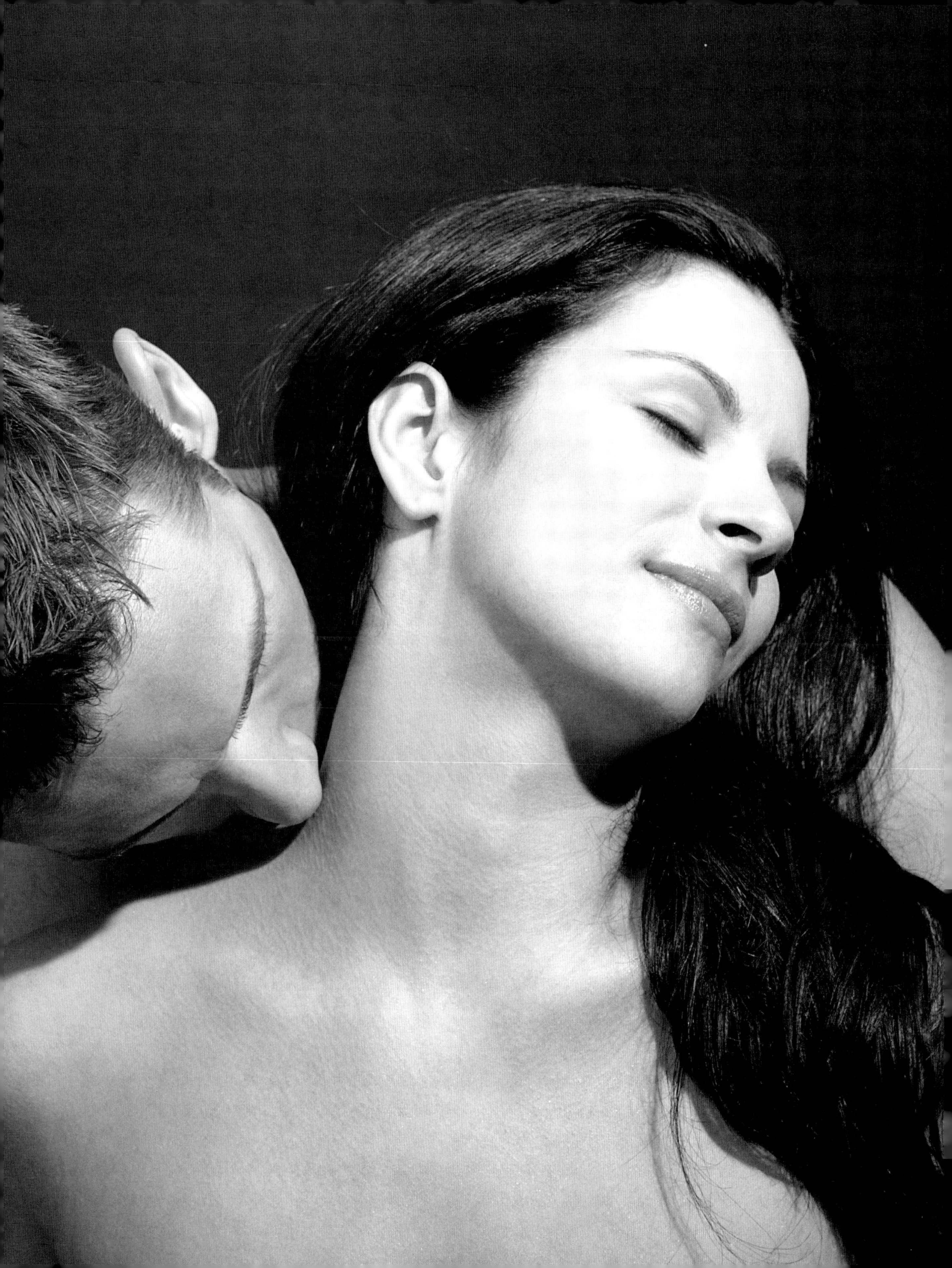

Scents That Turn Us On

Which scents provoke the greatest response? Because our sense of smell is processed in the part of the brain that governs emotions and memories, scent is the most personal of preferences. However, studies have been done that provide us with some intriguing indications. Alan R. Hirsch, M.D., neurological director of the Smell and Taste Treatment and Research Foundation in Chicago, found that the smell of cheese pizza increased blood flow to the penis by 5 percent, buttered popcorn by 9 percent, and lavender and pumpkin pie each by 40 percent. For women, lavender and pumpkin pie also had a stimulating effect; however, the smell of licorice combined with the scent of cucumber created the greatest increase in blood flow to the vagina. (These findings could certainly revolutionize the concept of a romantic dinner!) In comparison, floral perfume prompted only a 3-percent increase in blood flow to the penis among men. Among women, the smell of men's cologne actually lowered blood flow to the vagina. However, this study addresses only the physical aspect of arousal. The emotional component is much more individual.

I'm sure you've had the experience of smelling something that immediately took you back to another time and place. You probably experienced some of the same emotions you had felt at that time. This programming is powerful, but it can also be quite subtle. For example, you might find yourself unexpectedly turned off by someone you had previously found magnetic if he were to wear the same cologne as an unfaithful ex-boyfriend. Your conscious mind might not remember the fragrance, but the scent is indelibly embedded in your unconscious. It won't matter how many books recommend a certain fragrance as a sexual stimulant. If you don't like its smell, or the scent reminds you of something negative from your past, you won't be aroused.

You can use smell to program arousal. If both you and your partner like sandalwood, for example, and you light a stick of sandalwood incense every time you make love, it won't take long before you will become aroused anytime (and anywhere) you smell sandalwood.

Identify Your Favorites

Do you know for sure which scents turn you on? Write a list of your top five favorite scents. You can be attracted to the smell of just about anything. For example, one of my favorite aromas is the smell of a stable—the aroma of fresh hay mixed with the odor of horse (yes, including manure). I grew up adoring horses and even the scent of a well-worn saddle is still powerfully arousing to me. If you have trouble identifying your favorite scents, close your eyes and take a few deep breaths. Don't try too hard; just let the memories of yummy smells waft gently through your mind. Once you have your top five favorites, make another list of five smells that absolutely turn you off. Number one on my turnoff list is the smell of bananas. I can become seriously nauseated if someone unpeels a banana clear across the room. Another one of my top five turnoffs is licorice, even though research shows that most women find it a powerful turnon. Make your own list and do not judge yourself for your choices. Keep adding to and subtracting from this list as your tastes change. Share this list with your partner (it is a great getting-to-know-you game to play with a new partner) and ask him or her to tell you his or her preferences.

Traditional Aphrodisiacs

Historically, there are specific scents that are believed to elicit sexual response. If you don't like any of these scents, obviously they will not be arousing for you. But if you aren't familiar with some of these, give them a try. You may find yourself erotically surprised by their effect. (Note: If you are going to sample several scents in a row, sniff some roasted coffee beans between scents to clear your nose.)

MUSK is an animal scent, originally derived from the now nearly extinct musk deer. Other musk scents have been procured from civets and beavers. Ambergris is another precious musk produced by whales. Musk may be worn by both men and women.

SANDALWOOD is culled from trees that must be at least thirty years old. In India the wood is so precious it is reserved for sacred uses, such as construction of temples. Sandalwood is said to be able to transform sex into a spiritual experience. Its aroma aids creativity, intuition, serenity, meditation, and wisdom. It is traditionally recommended for men as a perfume but is equally good for men and women in all its other applications.

PATCHOULI has a reputation as a strong aphrodisiac. Some say that it stimulates the production of the feel-good hormones, endorphins. It is a scent reminiscent of the earth—deep humid rain forests and damp rich soil. Patchouli provides people with a sense of grounding: a comfort in their bodies and an intimacy with themselves. It is a scent often favored by the young and by natural rebels. Its euphoric and liberating qualities make it a perfect scent for passionate encounters of all kinds. Warning: The scent is strong and can linger for days, and the aroma is so distinctive that people generally either love it or hate it. Experiment with small quantities before overindulging.

YLANG-YLANG is considered a potent aphrodisiac. The ylang-ylang aroma can be soothing, act as an anti-depressant, and create a relaxing atmosphere. It calms anger and transforms negative emotions into positive feelings and sexual desire. It is considered a feminine scent, in that it allows men and women to express the feminine side of their natures. In Indonesia, its flower petals are often strewn across the marriage bed as a symbol of love. Its perfume liberates the sweetness of emotions. Like all passionate scents, it can be powerful, so use sparingly to avoid headaches.

ROSE Since ancient times, the rose has consistently been the archetype of love, femininity, and emotional feeling. Its fragrance clears the mind and evokes a feeling of well-being, harmony, and security. Rose has an affinity with the heart, allowing it to infuse our thoughts and actions with love. The aroma of rose harmonizes the sacred and the sensual aspects of sex. Rose is thought to be the preferred fragrance of the angels and a true expression of angelic nature.

JASMINE is the "queen of the night," so named because its flowers do not release their scent during the day. The Sufis revere jasmine as a symbol of both romantic and spiritual love. In the Hindu tradition, Kama, the god of love, tipped his arrows with jasmine flowers so they would have the power to infuse the heart with desire. Jasmine is euphoric and stimulates the hypothalamus to produce enkephalin, a substance that not only inhibits pain but provokes a state of well-being and happiness. Jasmine dissolves the fears and the tensions related to sexuality and is said to relieve impotence.

BERGAMOT, the familiar aroma of Earl Grey tea, is an invigorating scent. Its effects can range from inspirational to arousing. It's also known to clear the head and soothe grief. Bergamot mixes well with many other passionate scents.

FRANKINCENSE possesses extraordinary antiseptic properties and is purifying for both our homes and our minds. It also heightens awareness and stimulates the senses, making it a nice scent to use at the beginning of lovemaking. Try a blend of frankincense and ylang-ylang.

VANILLA is another good scent for the start of a passionate night. It typically appeals to both men and women. Vanilla is more of a feel-good scent than a stimulating one—perfect for easing the tensions and changing the mood at the end of a long, hard day.

NEROLI is the name of an essential oil distilled from the flowers of the bitter orange tree. The scents of both neroli and orange are associated with romance and sensuality. In many traditions, orange-blossom water is sprinkled on the heads of a bride and a groom, or they are crowned with orange blossoms. The aroma of orange and neroli increases physical and psychic energy and promotes feelings of joy.

Other plant scents that have been used as aphrodisiacs—either by themselves or in combination with other scents—include sage, clary sage, anise, fennel, angelica, geranium, cardamom, cinnamon, nutmeg, cypress, pine, and spruce. However, any scent you love can be used as an aphrodisiac. Do not be shy or embarrassed about what turns you on. I know people who are turned on by the smell of blood, mud, motor oil, and—you guessed it—leather.

Erotic Pulse Points

Anoint the body with scent at the pulse points:

a. **The temporal artery,** located between the tragus (that's the little piece of cartilage at the front of the ear opening) and the jaw.

b. **The carotid artery,** located at the front of the neck between the voice box and adjacent muscle.

c. **The subclavian artery,** located behind the clavicle, or collarbone. This may be a little tricky to find. Reach down inside the top edge of your collarbone and press down to feel the pulse.

d. **The radial artery,** the traditional pulse-taking point, located on the thumb side of the wrist.

e. **The brachial artery,** the point at which blood pressure is measured. It is on the inside of the arm, at the elbow and below the biceps on the little-finger side of the tendon that runs down the center of the arm.

f. **The popliteal artery,** located behind the knee.

Incorporate Scents Slowly and Mindfully

Whatever your preferences in scents, the key to the passionate possibilities of aroma is in how you use them. First and most important, start lightly. A scent that isalluring when applied sparingly can be nauseating when it's poured on. When you start with small amounts, it's possible to stop and clear the air or wash the scent off if you don't like it. Keep in mind that the art of luxurious loving encourages us to pay attention to what we really like. A scent that's simply not bad or just a bit too much is not good enough. Keep experimenting until you find a scent—or a blend of scents —that makes you melt.

I use the highest-quality incense and essential oils I can afford. Cheap incense and synthetic oils may contain unpleasant ingredients that can cause allergic reactions. An essential oil is a highly concentrated, aromatic oil extracted from the flowers, leaves, wood, or grass parts of plants. On an etheric level, essential oils carry a plant's soul.

Do not surprise your partner with a scent (unless, of course, that's the game you've agreed to play). Make sure he has a chance to sniff it before you use it in the room or apply it to either your body or his. Do not assume that a fragrance you like is going to appeal to your partner just because he loves you.

You can luxuriate in the aphrodisiacal magic of scents in any number of ways, including the following:

1. Light a stick of incense.
2. Put a drop of essential oil onto a hot lightbulb—incandescent, not halogen—or on the top of a candle.
3. Diffuse an essential oil in an aromatherapy burner.

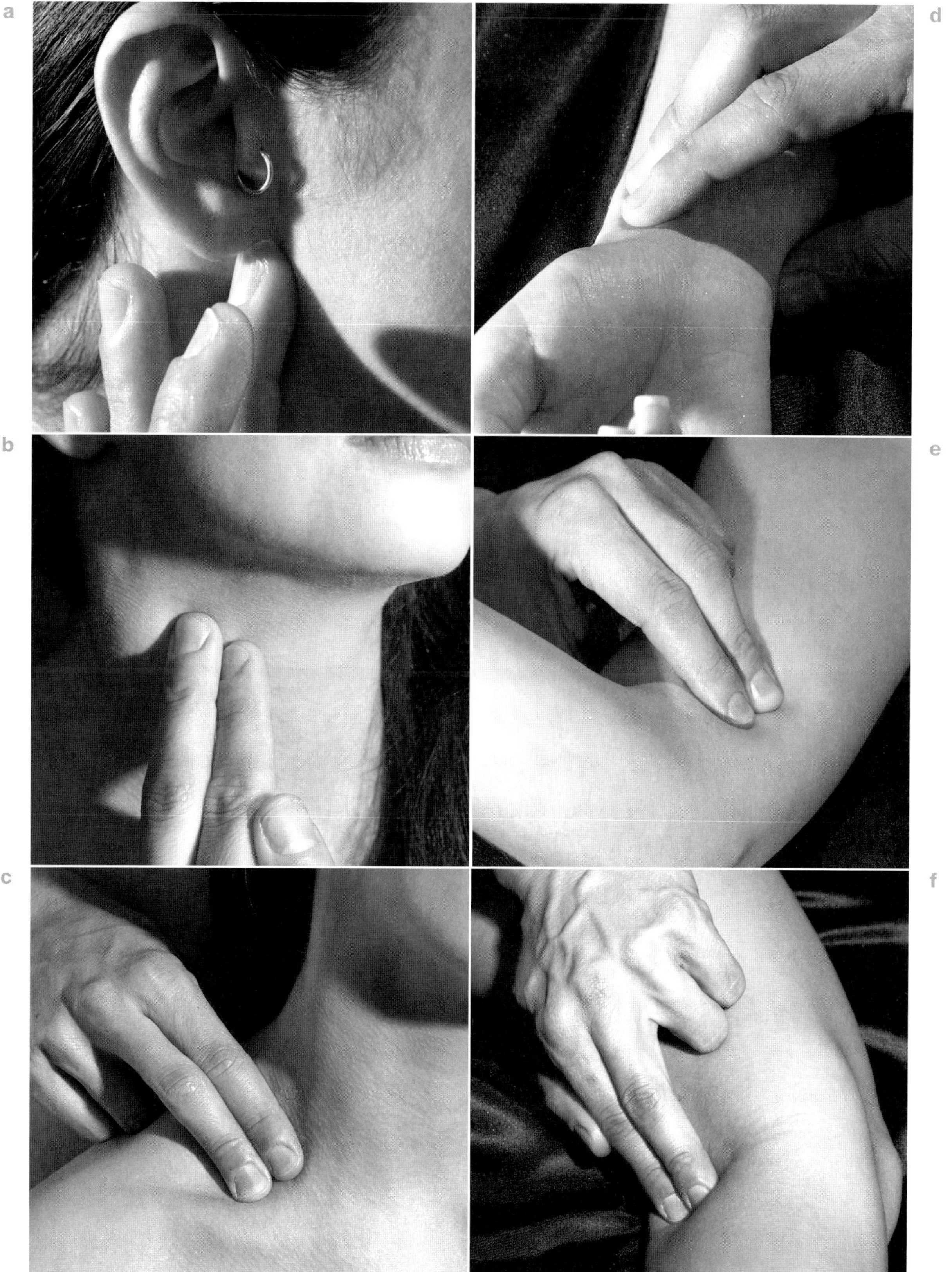
a
d
b
e
c
f

Put a few drops of oil and a small amount of water into the bowl of the burner and light the candle beneath.

4. Put a few drops of essential oil into a spray bottle of water and spritz the room—or your partner.
5. Make your own aromatic combinations. Mix two drops of one oil with three drops of another and five drops of a third. Write down your recipes so you can remember the ones you like best. When you find a combination you love, be sure to repeat it. The more you use the scent, the more you program it into your unconscious erotic mind. The effect is exponential; you will find yourself more and more turned on by it.

My favorite use of scent is on the body. I like to anoint myself with oils as a kind of self-blessing. I also enjoy anointing a partner or having a lover anoint me. There are specific points on the body that amplify scent best, specifically the pulse points, where arteries come close to the skin. When using scent on the body in more than one or two locations, you may prefer to dilute the essential oil with a few drops of unscented oil to avoid olfactory overload. You may anoint yourself, or your lover may anoint you with a drop of scented oil on any of the pulse points.

In an ancient Indian sex ritual, "The Rite of the Five Essentials," a woman was anointed with five oils on different parts of her body to lift her spirits so she might manifest as a goddess. Jasmine was applied to her hands, patchouli to her neck and cheeks, amber or musk to her breasts. Spikenard (an aromatic root stalk in the same family as Indian valerian) was rubbed into her hair, and sandalwood onto her thighs. You can create your own version of this ritual, applying your five favorite fragrances to the pulse points of your own god or goddess.

Other scent amplification spots on the body are the perspiration points, places where heat builds up and sends out a scent. You can perfume these points as well. They are between the breasts, the groin, and under the arms.

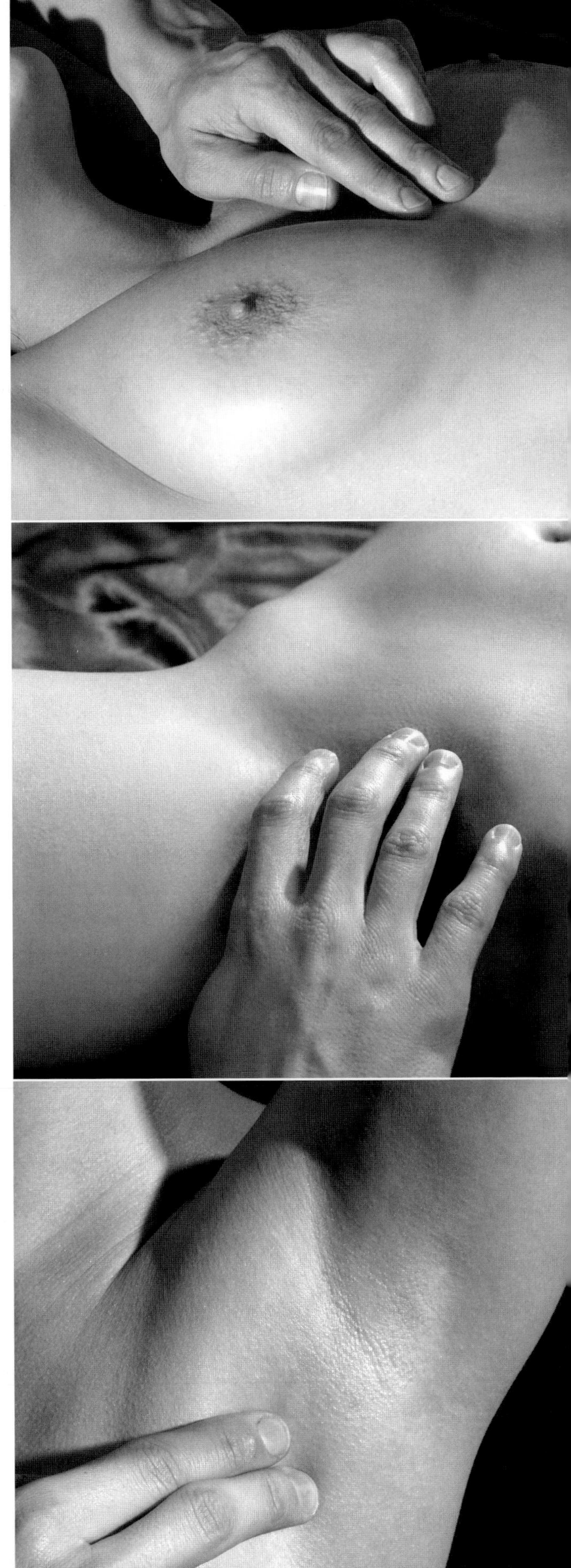

Rediscover Your Natural Scents

Speaking of perspiration, fresh—not stale—perspiration is a proven aphrodisiac. Each person has an odor print as unique as the fingerprint. This is influenced by a number of variables, including diet, gender, heredity, health, medication, and mood. Odor is a communication system we are usually unaware of. It's a statement about who we are, and even what emotional state we are in. For instance, when adrenaline is produced by the adrenal glands, it actually changes your odor. That is why animals are actually able to smell fear. A similar phenomenon happens during sex. Haven't you noticed that when you are in the throes of passionate sex with a lover you adore, you are turned on by her sweat? This may have something todo with those mysterious chemicals called pheromones. Pheromones, manufactured by the apocrine (sweat) glands, are odiferous substances chemically similar to hormones that are secreted by endocrine glands.

The word *pheromone* is from the Greek *pherein*—to carry—and *hormon*—to excite. In the animal world, pheromones are individual scent "prints" found in urine or sweat that dictate sexual behavior and attract the opposite sex. They help animals identify one another and choose a mate with an immune system different enough from their own to ensure healthy offspring. Animals have a special organ in their noses called the vomeronasal organ (VNO) that detects this odorless chemical.

A human VNO has also been found in some, but not all, people. The VNO is part of the nasal system but is independent of smell, so you cannot actually smell pheromones. Nevertheless, studies have shown that even though modern humans are overwhelmingly visually oriented when it comes to choosing a partner, pheromones are alluring and do play a part in human sexual response. Human pheromones are most densely concentrated in sweat, skin, and hair. When we slow down our lovemaking and take the time to appreciate our partner's unique, exciting scent, our arousal levels can rise dramatically.

Try this: Right after your partner gets out of the bath or shower—before she has applied any perfume, sniff her. That's right, sniff your partner all over. The warm moisture of freshly washed skin holds a bouquet of aromas. (If you prefer, you can also try this *before* she gets into the shower.) Close your eyes and start at the top of her head. What do you smell? Perhaps a hint of the shampoo she used? Move down to her face and neck. Another scent? Perhaps of her face soap? Now move down her body for a third scent. Our scent changes in different places on our body. You will recognize your lover's unique scent, regardless of any scent her bath products may have left lingering on her skin. If you are the one doing the sniffing, go into it totally. Try to *become* the scent of your lover. Attempt to inhale her so deeply that she becomes part of you. If you have trouble letting go enough to really experience the delight of your lover's aroma, pretend you are a puppy, exploring a species of mammal you have never encountered before. If you are the one being sniffed, relax. Breathe. Let yourself be inhaled. Eventually, the sniffing may get so intense it becomes ticklish. You may both dissolve in a heady, breath-and-scent-induced fit of giggles. Enjoy it! When your giggles subside, notice your arousal level. You may want to continue with more lovemaking, or you may feel completely satisfied with your nosegasm.

OPPOSITE The perspiration points also amplify fragrance: between the breasts, the groin, under the arm.

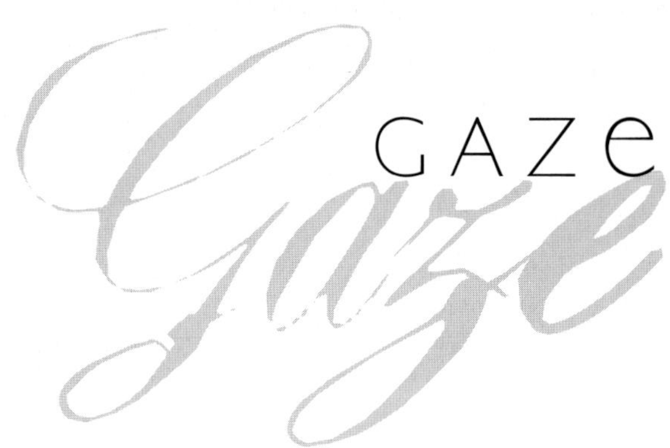

GAZE

4

EVERYTHING WE VIEW THROUGH THE lens of Eros either turns us on, turns us off, or has a neutral effect. When we first fall in love, everything we see about our partner turns us on—the way he looks, the way he moves, his hands, his hair, his eyes—every square inch of him is delicious. We spend hours thinking of our lover and how we can make ourselves more attractive for him. When we are with him, we spend hours gazing into his eyes.

When we fall in love, the human body produces a cocktail of love chemicals. Dopamine produces a feeling of bliss. Norepinephrine, similar to adrenaline, produces a racing heart and a feeling of excitement. Together, these two chemicals produce euphoria, intense energy, sleeplessness, loss of appetite, and sharply focused attention. Further compounding the effect, researchers have found that the sight of our lover —either in person or in a photograph—causes increased blood flow to the areas of the brain with receptors for dopamine, exponentially increasing our obsession with our beloved.

Over time, this chemical cocktail diminishes and by the time our relationship is two years old, levels have returned to their preobsession levels. Other chemicals, such as endorphins and oxytocin (which is released when you and your partner have sex), are still present. But the "love is blind" period is over. More and more of what we see about our partner has a neutral, rather than turn-on, effect. Unless we are in the middle of making love, we do not spend long stretches of time gazing into each other's eyes. It's not that we don't find our partner attractive and desirable, it's just that she has become a bit familiar. We tend to focus on what we already know about her. We rarely, if ever, expect to find something new. Similarly, we tend to overlook the ways in which we are growing and changing in relation to her. The remedy for this romantic malaise is to look at ourselves and our lover with new eyes.

In Tantra, it is said that the eyes are the gateway to the soul. After the love cocktail has worn off, eye gazing can almost seem too intimate unless we are very aroused.

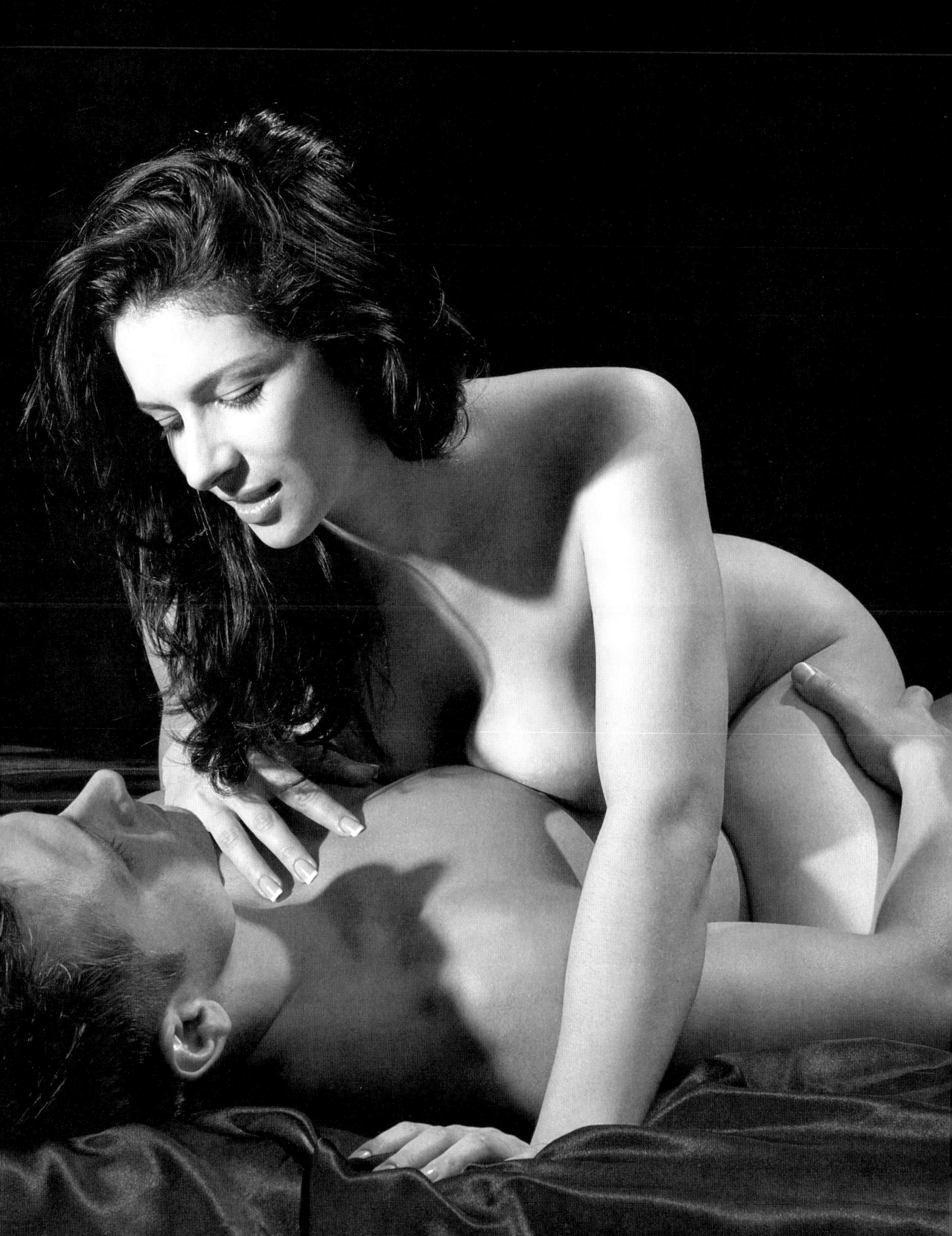

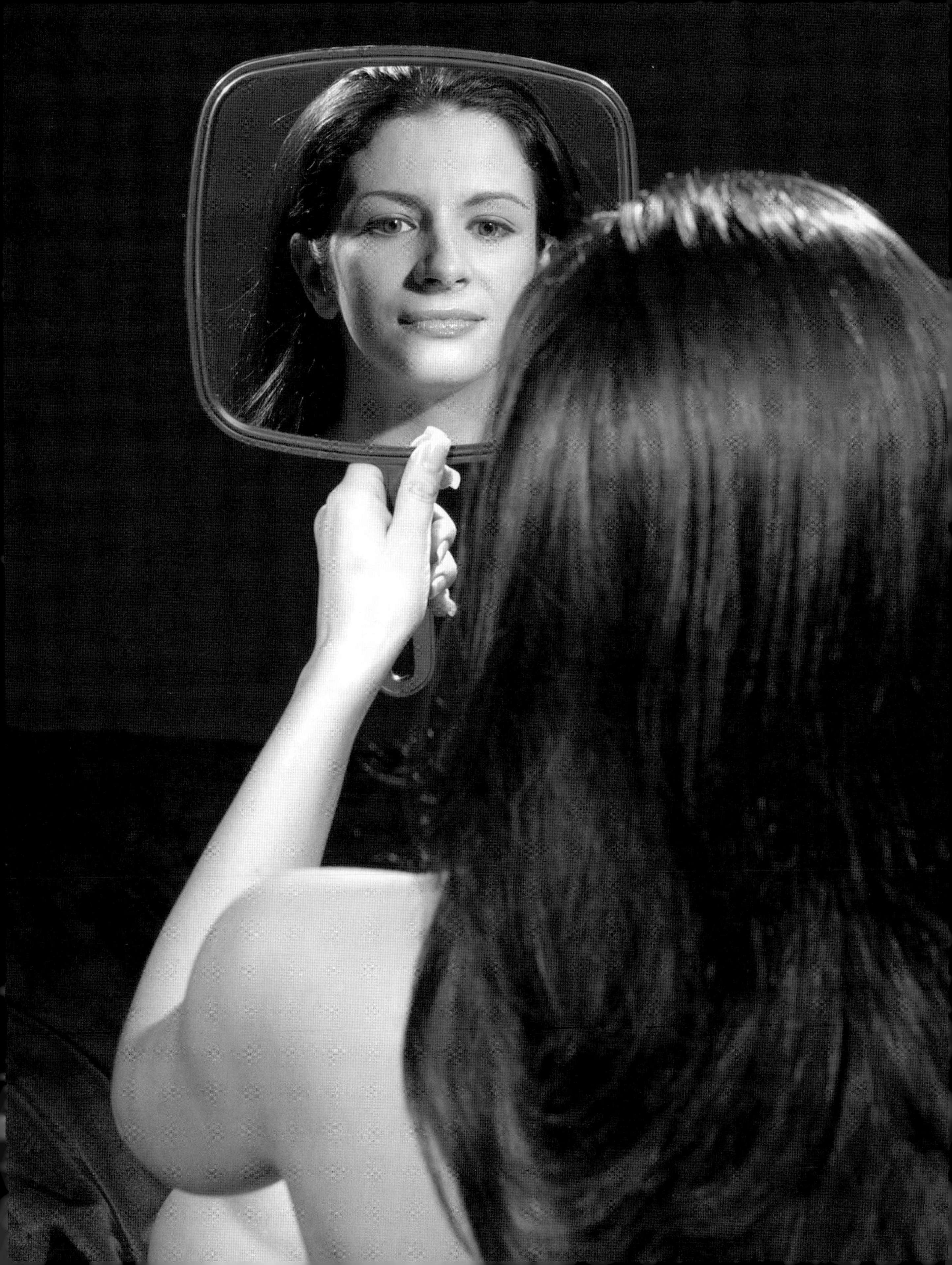

However, the mindful, deliberate practice of eye gazing—especially when we are about to make love—can lead to a new, deeper kind of intoxication and intimacy. Eye gazing is a trust exercise of the highest order. Before practicing it with your lover, try it with yourself.

Appreciate Yourself with Soft Eyes

Hold a hand mirror in one hand. Place your other hand on your heart. Look into the mirror and gaze into your own nondominant eye. (If you are right-handed, your left eye is your nondominant eye; if you are left-handed, it's your right eye.) Breathe. Maintain your gaze. Resist the temptation to criticize—or to even notice—wrinkles, blemishes, and unplucked eyebrows. Instead, imagine your eye as a pool that reveals your soul. Immerse yourself in that pool.

Look at yourself with "soft eyes." To understand how this works, first stare into the mirror looking directly at the pupil of your nondominant eye. Now "soften" your eyes, still looking into the mirror but not staring so hard. Did you notice how your peripheral vision opened up and how you were able to see more with less effort? Are you less judgmental when looking at yourself this way?

Now try some appreciation. As you eye gaze with yourself with soft eyes, speak out loud—or silently if speaking makes you uncomfortable—some words of appreciation for yourself. You might compliment yourself on your beautiful eyes, on your courage, or on your compassion. This may be challenging, as we are not encouraged to praise ourselves, especially out loud. But keep going. When we are able to look into our own eyes and speak loving words, we become more open and compassionate with a partner. The power of eye gazing is so strong it has even been measured scientifically. A university professor put unacquainted men and women together for ninety minutes and had them discuss intimate details about themselves. Then he told them to stare into each other's eyes for four minutes without talking. After the experiment, many of the subjects felt a deep attraction for their partner and six months later, two of them got married.

OPPOSITE When we are able to look into our own eyes and speak loving words, we become more open and compassionate with a partner.

Share an Intimate Gaze with Your Partner

If eye gazing can be that powerful between strangers, imagine what it can do between lovers committed to extended states of pleasure. Just before you next make love, try eye gazing in this Tantric-inspired position: Sit across from your partner with your legs crossed comfortably. Place your right hand over your partner's heart. Your partner places her right hand over your heart. Now place your left hand over your partner's right hand (which is on your heart). Your partner places her left hand over your right hand (which is on her heart). Breathe together and look into each other's left (or nondominant) eye. Allow a sigh or "ahhh" to come out every four or five breaths or so. Continue for thirty or forty breaths, or until you feel your hearts open and connected. This exercise helps you both feel safe and reconnect with your partner.

Over the course of an intimate long-term relationship, it is natural to feel some disconnection. That does not mean you have stopped loving your partner or he you. It is natural, healthy, and, in fact, desirable for two people to maintain their sense of individuality apart

OPPOSITE Eye gazing with a partner reawakens intimacy and desire.

from their partner. When two happy, self-satisfied, self-loving people come together out of a sense of desire, not need, the resulting relationship is a thriving one. Over time and given the demands of busy lives, more separation may occur than you would like. Eye gazing and looking at each other with new, soft eyes will reawaken intimacy and desire.

One of the rewards of making love mindfully is the ability to cease any negative internal self-talk about not being physically attractive enough. We may be embarrassed by all manner of body imperfections, from size to scars to stretch marks. Our lovers may tell us that we are gorgeous, hot, and desirable, but we just can't believe that they could mean that, when we know we've put on ten pounds in the past two months and our cellulite is getting worse. Women in particular have a distorted view of what the female body is supposed to look like. Men can have a similarly skewed view of their bodies. In addition to the pumped-up, airbrushed images we see in the media every day, childhood memories play a part in how good or bad we think we look. For example, if you were always ashamed of an obese parent, you may think that the five pounds you gained over the holidays make you look more like that parent. This kind of embarrassment and discomfort with our bodies takes away not only our pleasure at being seen by our lover but also his pleasure at seeing us. Everyone's idea of beauty is different. Even before your lover first spoke to you, he was attracted to you because you fit his idea of beautiful. To your lover, your nude body is hot. When he looks at you, he is not critiquing you, he is desiring you. Try to see and love your body the way your lover does.

SENSUOUS UNDRESSING

One way to do this is with a little game called Sensuous Undressing. Stand with feet hip distance apart in a comfortably warm, candlelit room. Close your eyes. Let your partner undress you as slowly as possible. He appreciates each and every square inch of your body as he slowly reveals it. You drop into the sensation of being sensuously undressed and worshiped. If you are doing the undressing, remove each garment as though it were a jewel-covered piece of silk. Breathe. Go s-l-o-w-l-y. Appreciate every curve and detail of this beautiful body. Show your lover your appreciation by gently stroking each newly uncovered body part. If you are being undressed, breathe. Do not help your lover undress you. If he needs to move your arm, he will. If he needs to raise your foot, he will. Just receive the undressing. Feel the love and reverence in his touch.

While you are undressing your partner, you may notice that the closer you get to his body, the better it looks. Let's say your lover has a poochy tummy. When you look at him from across the room, you notice the tummy. However, when you are in bed together, you are aware of only how beautiful his butt is or how the curve of his bicep is so strong and hot. Imperfections—real or perceived—vanish. Exercises such as Sensuous Undressing keep the focus close-up, where all bodies look delicious. And remember, your lover loves your body just the way it is. He or she will be aware of only the things you dislike about it if you keep obsessing about them! Stop criticizing your body right now.

THINK OF YOUR BODIES AS ART

You can learn to love your body sensually and sexually by simply adorning it. I do not mean covering it up—I mean highlighting your best features. Do you have luscious breasts? Adorn your nipples with pasties or jewelry. Women-owned companies such as divadots.com or twirlygirl.net sell fun, unique adornments. If you've

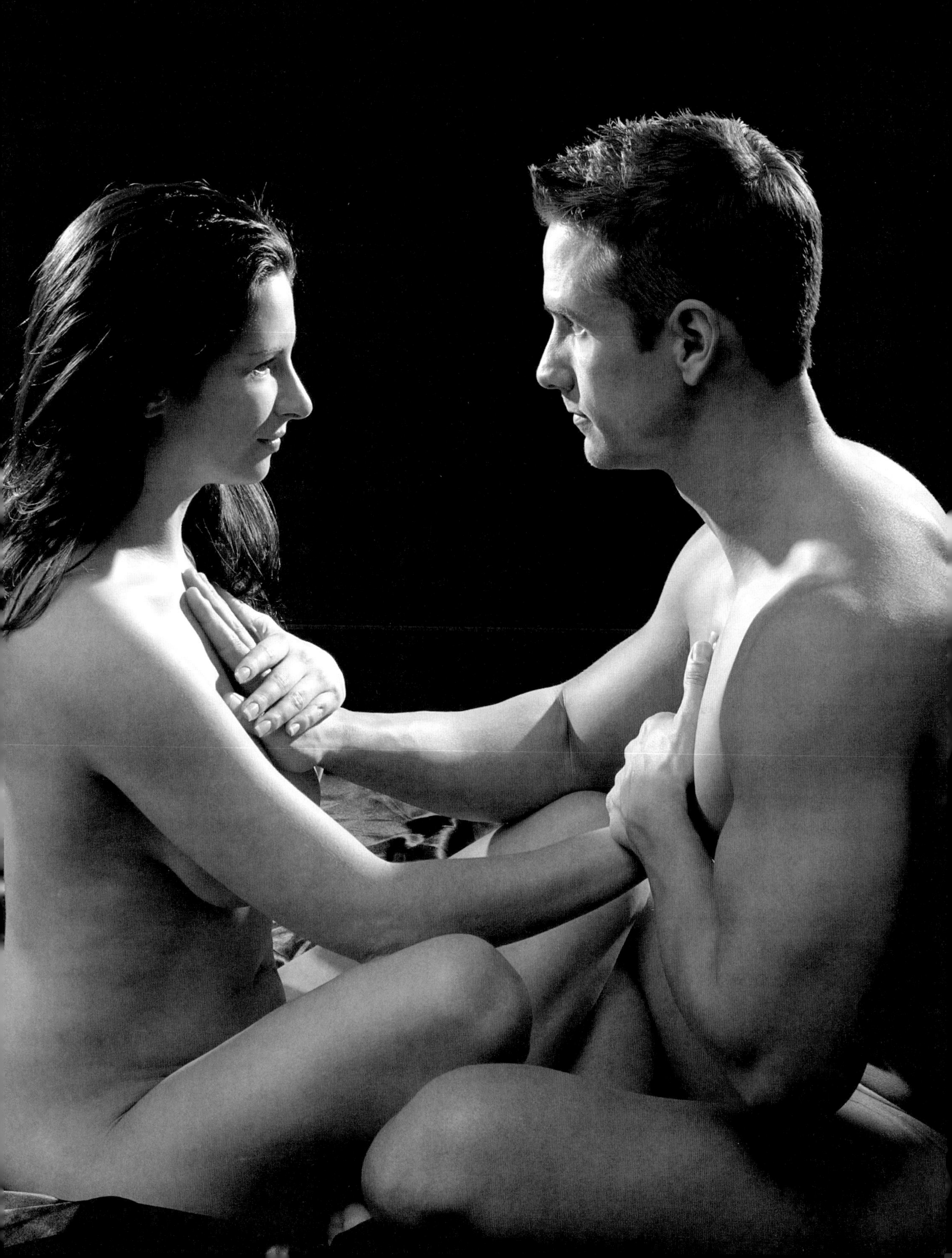

always liked the look of metal jewelry but can't imagine a nipple piercing, try pierceless nipple jewelry. Perhaps your best feature is your round firm derriere. Tie a semi-sheer silk sarong around your hips—this goes for men, too. Try alternating (or combining) soft, sheer fabrics with the harder feel of leather. Sexy leather garments are available in every cut and style imaginable and feel as sensuous to wear as theyare provocative to look at. Choose body adornments that make you look and feel sexy. If you are oozing self-love and self-lust, your partner will be attracted by that energy. It won't be the costume that turns her on, it will be you.

Appreciate your lover's body as the magnificent work of art it is by literally making it art. Paint it! You do not have to be a great artist, nor do you have to cover every square inch of flesh. You can paint on some lacy lingerie or a corset and stockings. Or some leopard spots or feathers or fins. You can paint abstract swirls that start at the neck and curve around the breast and follow the curve of the belly and buttocks. Or adorn them with powerful magic symbols. What you paint is less important than how you paint it. While you are creating a visual masterpiece, your partner will be being teased and stroked with your varied brushstrokes. Do not start with the most obvious erogenous zones. Build up the excitement. Tease. (Suggestions for erogenous zones you might want to decorate can be found in chapter 9, "Caress.") Vary the sensations you produce by varying your tools. Use artist's brushes, sponges, cotton swabs, feathers, the tip of a rosebud, and your fingers. Each will produce unique sensations and designs. A water-soluble acrylic craft paint is your best choice. It is nonirritating to most skin types and washes off easily. You can also use finger-paint bath soap and glow-in-the-dark paint, both of which can be found in toy stores or the children's section of a drugstore. Some adventurous lovers like to paint their lovers' hands or feet with henna. Henna tattoos, such as the ones Indian brides apply to their hands and feet prior to wedding ceremonies, are semipermanent. It takes from a few days to a few weeks for these to fade, so proceed accordingly. Henna tattooing kits are readily available online and in many beauty-supply stores. Heighten your partner's sensuous enjoyment while you are turning her body into a masterpiece by blindfolding her. Tell her that you are a temperamental artist who refuses to let her see his canvas until it is complete. When she can't see, your lover's sense of touch is heightened dramatically, along with her imagination.

Keep It Playful Remember to breathe while you are painting and being painted. Relax your shoulders. This is not an art class and you are not being judged. You are indulging in the childlike activity of painting! Your intention is to have fun and give your partner pleasure. If you keep a sense of playfulness and adventure, you and your partner will both feel deliciously altered by the time your painting is finished. You may want to document your artwork with pictures. If body painting becomes a favorite sensuous activity, you could build up your own personal erotic-art gallery. Erotic photography is a wonderful way to get over thinking of yourself as not sexy or beautiful enough. Being photographed during sex may sound strange, but it can be very exciting and build a huge amount of sexual energy. Let your partner photograph you during various stages of arousal. Everyone looks beautiful when turned on. Have you ever secretly fantasized about posing for *Playboy* or *Playgirl*? Or have you ever thought about being the cameraperson for an erotic movie? We all have an inner exhibitionist and an inner voyeur. You can often tell which of these personalities is dominant by what people do for a living. Photographers and documentary filmmakers are natural voyeurs. Actors and dancers are natural exhibitionists. Which are you? Depending on the day and the circumstances, you may be both!

Keep It Mindful If you are at all shy about this, start slowly. Tell your partner your limits—for example, no genital shots, orgasm shots, or no more than three photos. And, of course, the person being photographed "owns" the photos and can either trash them or frame them. If you are the photographer, think of the camera as a sex toy. Remember your intention. How would you use the camera if your intention were not to get the world's most perfect picture but to turn your lover on? If your intention were to get a gorgeous picture of your lover in order to show her how beautiful she is to you, you would use the camera differently. If you are being photographed, you can also have an intention. Your intention may be to let your inner exhibitionist go wild. Or you may simply want to see what you look like making love. Breathe! Make believe that each camera click or flash is like a tongue licking your clitoris or a luscious mouth sinking down on your cock. Make love to that camera!

Focus Your Fantasies

Our eyes are not the only portal through which we see. Our imagination is one of our richest sources of visual information and inspiration. One very pleasurable use of our imagination is fantasy, especially sexual fantasy. Sexual fantasies are erotic stories we use to entertain our brain. They are also the rehearsal hall for new erotic experiences and new sexual possibilities. The mindful use of fantasy can be an intriguing and powerful complement to prolonged arousal and escalating pleasure. Conversely, the unconscious use of fantasy will take your focus off your body and your partner. Any fantasy that takes you out of the present moment will ultimately drain sexual energy away from your experience. Welcoming a willing lover into your fantasy allows you both to put your attention where your intentions are. Together you can build sexual energy. It is not the content of your sexual fantasy that makes it mindful—it's how you use it. All your sexual fantasies are healthy—even the darkest, filthiest, most violent ones. Think of your imagination as a big powerful movie studio. Hundreds of story ideas come in daily. It is up to you—the head of the studio—to decide which ideas get written into scripts and then made into movies. Some stories will become award-winning pictures. Some will never see the light of day. But most of the stories that you read contain at least a snippet of a good idea that may inspire a great scene. If movie studios refused to accept all story ideas because they were afraid of seeing some bad ones, very few movies would ever get made. Similarly, when we censor our "inappropriate" fantasies, we may miss inspired erotic opportunities. For example, you may like to fantasize about forced sex, sex with a stranger, having a penis instead of a vagina (or vice versa), being paid for sex or having sex in public. You may or may not actually want to try any of these in real life. Yet all of them are ripe with real-life erotic possibilities. Examine your fantasies for elements you'd like to physic-alize. You might like to be put in light bondage with a blindfold and earplugs so that your sense of touch is magnified a hundredfold. You might like to pretend for an evening that you and your lover are strangers as you enjoy the ritual of discovering each other's bodies for the first time. You may want to make love outdoors at night with the risk of being discovered. These are all fantasy-inspired possibilities that can become powerful new opportunities for sexual expansion. Make time to explore your own erotic imagination. If you almost always run the same fantasy in your mind as you masturbate, then deliberately create

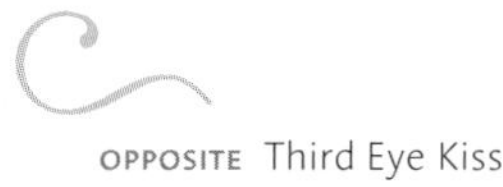

OPPOSITE Third Eye Kiss

a new one. In fact, if you always fantasize while you masturbate, practice not fantasizing. Keep your focus on the sensations your body is experiencing. Your body has its own imagination, and getting lost in sensation will open your body and your mind to new sexual possibilities.

Your eyes not only take in erotically stimulating images, they also move sexual energy around your body. The erotic meditation in chapter 2 ("Breathe") demonstrates how to use your breath to bring orgasmic energy up to your heart. You can similarly use your eyes to bring sexual energy up to the top of your head. With your eyelids closed, first look directly ahead, then roll your eyes up as though you could look out through the top of your head. This eye movement happens spontaneously during orgasm, but doing it consciously while you are charging your body with sexual energy stretches the lateral muscles of your eyes. This produces bursts of alpha waves in the brain, and that can lead to some very pleasant moments of trance and altered consciousness.

THE THIRD EYE

In the Tantric tradition, you have a Third Eye, a nonphysical eye located on your forehead between your eyebrows. This eye sees the invisible—your intuitions, insights, and visions. These are not the same as those gut hunches you feel about whether or not something is safe or dangerous but, rather, those inspi-rations that feel like the calling of your soul. Through your Third Eye you can see just who you are. You see the nature of your true calling. The visions seen through this eye nourish your uniqueness and your ecstatic nature. Sending sexual energy to this area intensifies those visions.

When you are eye gazing with your lover, you are using not only your physical eyes but also your Third Eye. Even when you close your eyelids, your Third Eye is open. Utilize this connection as you are building sexual energy. When you breathe your sexual energy up from your genitals into your Third Eye, you may see colors or feel it pulsing. Join with your lover in a Third Eye Kiss. With your physical eyes open, "kiss" with your foreheads. Breathe deeply. Let this be a long kiss. You may feel as if you and your lover are melting together. You may see visions. You may feel you are plugged into a powerful energy source. You are, in fact, tapped into the heavenly realm of erotic bliss.

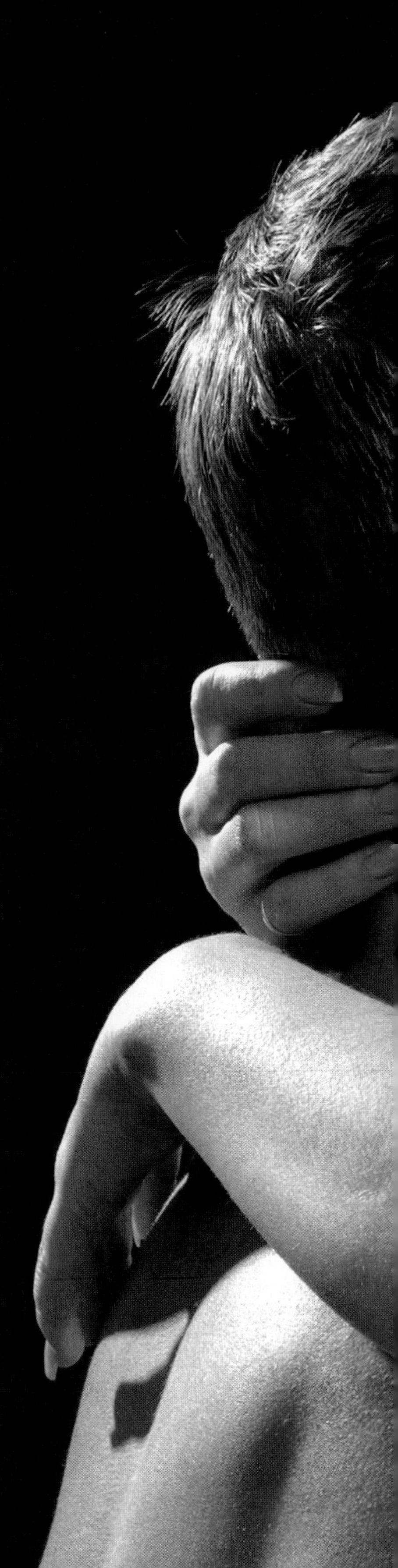

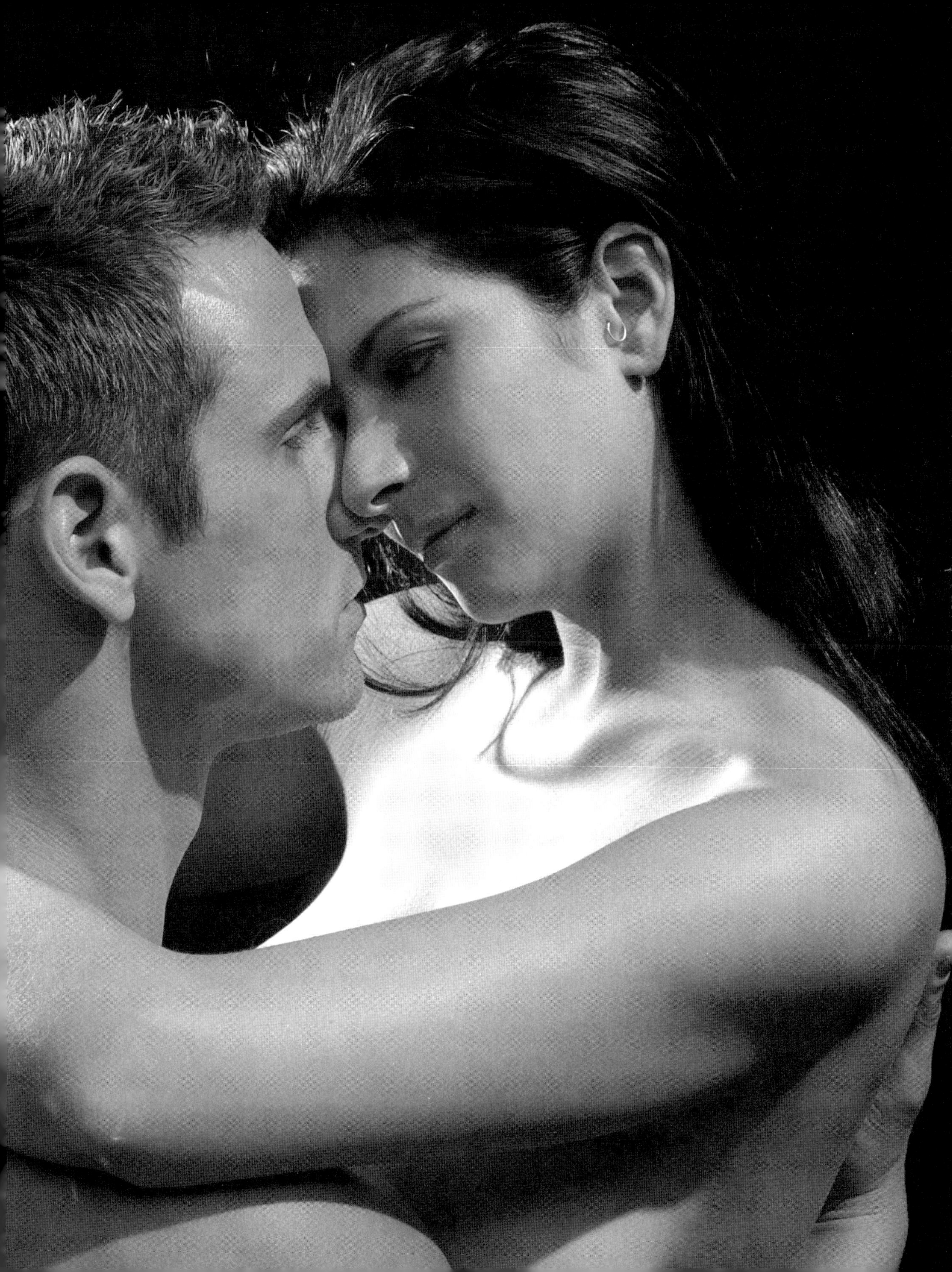

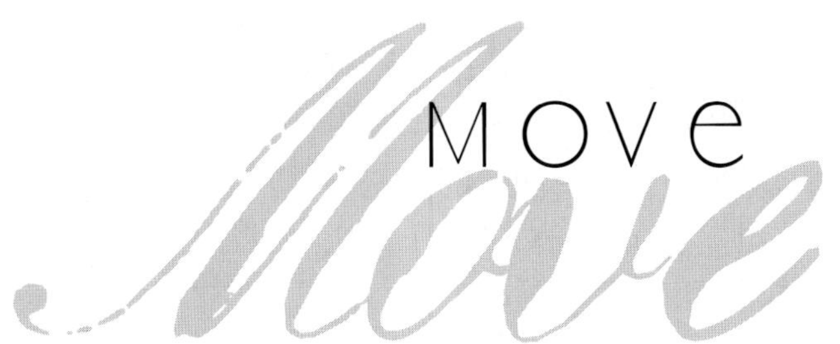

Move

5

TRY THIS LITTLE GAME: TELL YOUR lover to lie back and encourage her to remain motionless while you pleasure her. Tease her. Kiss her all over. Suck her earlobe, stroke the inside of her thigh. Massage her breasts and kiss her deeply. Every time she moves, stop what you are doing until she is perfectly still again. Then continue. Unless your partner is the world's most accomplished submissive, it will be impossible for her to remain completely still while you use every one of your erotic talents to arouse her. She will move, if only inside. Her breath will quicken, her vaginal walls will expand, and her clitoris will pound with blood. She may shudder and vibrate to some inner rhythm. She may clutch the sheets to try to prevent her pelvis from rocking. She may not be able to keep her head from moving from side to side. In short, sex without movement is a superhuman effort. Sex is energy and energy is always in motion. Like the electrical current in your home, your sexual energy is always present, always running through your body. The difference is that when you turn off the light in your bedroom, the light in your kitchen does not get brighter. Happily, your body doesn't work that way. When you close down one avenue of sexual expression, the sexual energy you raise in your body is magnified and expressed in other ways. This is why many people find sensory-deprivation play so incredibly hot. For example, if your partner blindfolds you and puts earplugs in your ears, your sense of taste may become exquisitely acute. Placing your partner in bondage may greatly heighten her ability to sense movement within her body. She may feel as though her clitoris is three inches long and pounding like a drum. Or she may suddenly be able to hear the water flowing in the pipes in the walls. Sexual energy is always electrifying your body. The longer you build the energy, the more powerful and ecstatic your experience will be.

OPPOSITE The longer you build the energy, the more powerful and ecstatic your experience will be.

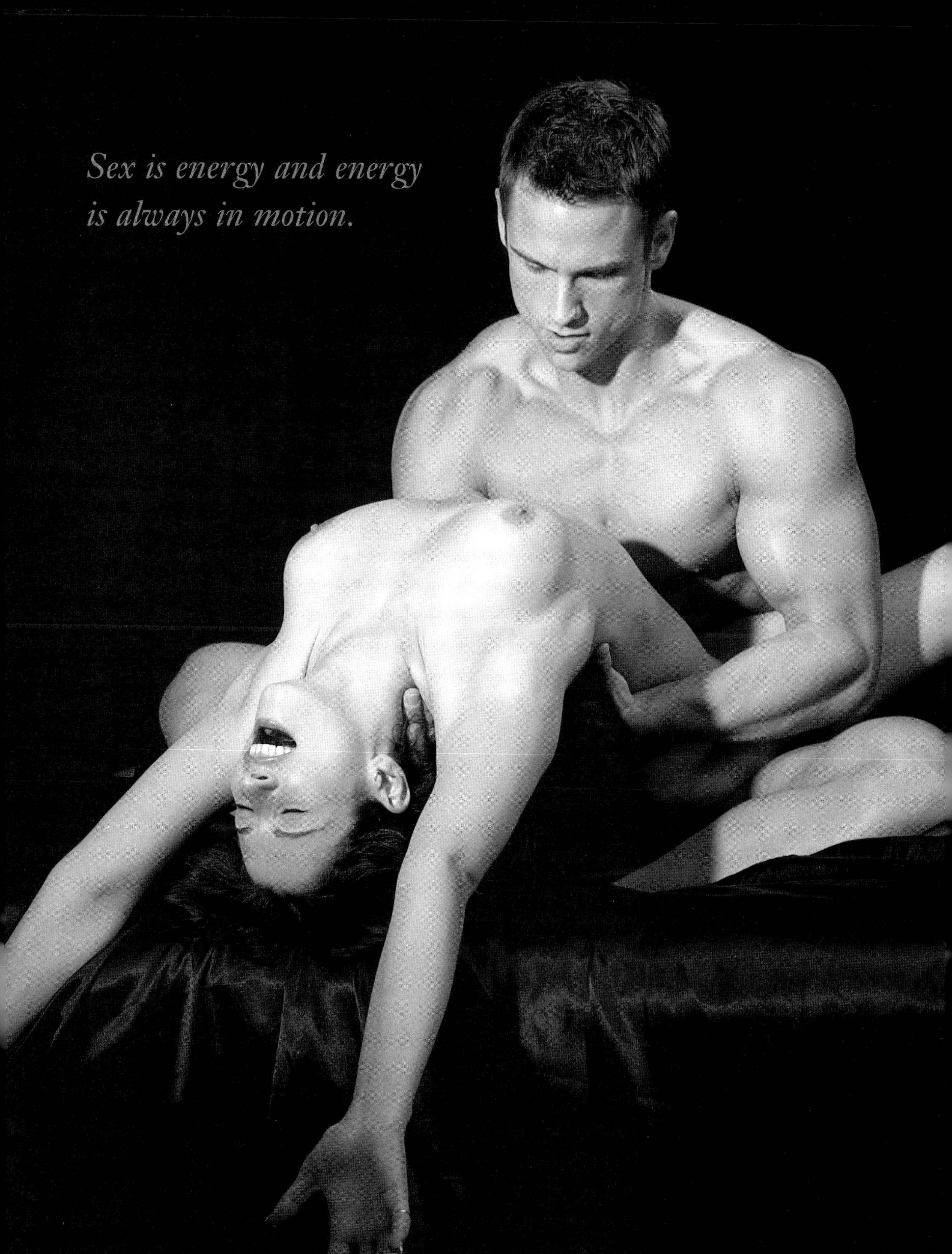

Sex is energy and energy is always in motion.

Movement Is Your Energy Generator for Sex

Not only does sexual energy cause your body to move but the reverse is also true. Movement is an essential energy generator in sex. The body wants to move. It shakes, undulates, contracts, expands, arches, rolls, twitches, shudders, tenses, and surrenders. Each instinctive response to arousal has a purpose—to build the sexual energy and move it throughout the body. However, we don't need to wait for sexual energy to make our pelvis gyrate or our back arch. We can consciously use all of sex's natural motions to build erotic heat in any part of the body. For example, during vaginal penetration, both men and women use their PC (pubococcygeus) muscles—the man in thrusting his penis, the woman in squeezing the penis. However, we can deliberately squeeze our PC muscle much earlier in the excitement phase of lovemaking to intensify our pleasure. Let's try that now.

DO KEGELS

First, find your PC muscle. Imagine you are in the bathroom peeing and someone unexpectedly opens the bathroom door. What do you do? You stop peeing. Feel that? That little muscle that stopped the flow of urine? That's the PC muscle. Give it a squeeze. That little contraction and release is called a Kegel. Kegels are your own personal erotic energy pumps. These little squeezes have been integral parts of sexual fitness and pleasure in many cultures for centuries. Kegels, when practiced regularly, tone and strengthen the PC muscle, making it easier for women to reach orgasm and to have stronger orgasms. The vagina grows more sensitive and the vaginal muscle becomes strong enough to massage a man's penis. (There will be more on this technique, called Pompoir, in chapter 10, "Connect.") Men who Kegel regularly will find that their erections are stronger and their orgasms are more intense. Kegels will also strengthen and tone the muscles involved in ejaculation, so men can gain greater control over the timing of their ejaculations. Both men and women will find that Kegels can be used in combination with just about any other sexual-energy-building technique to propel sexual energy throughout the body.

I recommend that you do one hundred to two hundred Kegels daily. You can Kegel while walking down the street or waiting for a traffic light to change, or while waiting in line at the cash machine. You can even use Kegels to spice up a boring business meeting. No one will know you are doing your sexercises.

Here is a simple round of Kegel exercises:

1. Gently squeeze the PC muscle for a couple of seconds.
   Release.
2. Squeeze. Release. Repeat for a total of eight Kegels.
3. Now do some Flutters—that's eight Kegels as fast as you can.
4. Do a second set of eight regular Kegels. Repeat the sequence.

Be gentle. If you're doubling over with each squeeze, you are working too hard! Don't worry if it feels as if you are also tightening your anus when you Kegel. That isn't a problem. But as you strengthen your PC muscle, you'll probably notice that you can isolate it more and more from the surrounding muscles.

While Kegels are especially efficient for moving sex-ual energy up the body once you are aroused, other types of movements are particularly suited to preparing your body to become aroused. When your intention is to stay in the arousal phase for as long as possible, sex becomes an erotic meditation. As in any meditation, a quiet mind is required to be able to focus on your body, on your partner, and on sensation. Mind chatter and galloping thoughts are unwelcome but inevitable distractions. The moment we try to slow down, all the thoughts that haven't been able to grab our attention rush in and start screaming, "Me! Me! Deal with me now!" Unpleasant as this is at any time, it is especially unwelcome when we want to get lost in pleasure with our beloved.

SHAKE

I use shaking as an active meditation technique that allows my natural crazy busy mind to speak and scream and worry and natter away, until finally my body and mind can come to a place of relaxation and energized awareness. Relaxed, energized awareness is precisely the state I would like to be in when I approach my beloved.

Try it. Shake. Just shake. Allow the shaking to start at your feet or in your hands and then travel up your body to the top of your head. You'll have to make an effort to get the shaking started, but after it gets moving, it will take on a life of its own. Eventually you won't have to shake; the shaking will shake you. Keep your eyes closed or use a blindfold. If you live in a small space and fear you'll crash into things, simply plant your feet on the floor in one spot and shake in place. Shake for fifteen to twenty minutes.

Now, I warn you, strange things may happen inside your head when you shake for this long. Every fear, worry, and preoccupation lurking in the darkest corners of your mind may come up demanding center stage. Try not to get carried away with any particular thought. Imagine lying on your back in a meadow on a breezy day, watching the clouds—in this case, your thoughts—float by. You simply notice that there are thoughts and what they look like. You don't jump on them and let them take you away. For example, you might find yourself thinking about money. Instead of allowing your mind to spend twenty minutes worrying about how you are going to pay your credit-card bill, you simply think, "Oh, look, here comes another terrifying thought about money. And there it goes. Bye-bye." You don't fight the thought or beat yourself up for having it, you just notice it and let it pass.

The experience of being shaken is very freeing. It brings warmth, aliveness, and even a tingling sensation…

An effective and fun way to help your partner loosen up his body and quiet his mind is to shake him. Have him stand with his feet hip distance apart with knees slightly bent. Shake his leg by putting your hands on either side of his calf and vibrating his calf muscle from side to side. Work your way up and shake his thigh. Then shake the other leg. Keep moving up his body. You can get a really good shaking going in the buttocks and it feels amazing. Using the same side-to-side vibrating technique, shake the belly and chest, then the lower and upper arms. You can also hold your partner's wrist in both of your hands and gently shake the whole arm. Just be sure not to put too much strain on the shoulder. You can even shake your partner's face for him! Be creative. What else can you shake? An earlobe? Fingers? Shoulders? The experience of being shaken is very freeing. It brings warmth, aliveness, and even a tingling sensation to body parts that may have gone numb under the stresses and strains of everyday life. It can also lead to giggles or even gales of laughter, which brings more energy to the festivities. Go with whatever happens. It's all good.

DANCE

Dancing can be a particularly erotic moving meditation that you can do with or without a partner. Approach dancing as you would the shaking meditation. Choose twenty minutes of music that makes you want to move, close your eyes, and let the dance dance you. Do not worry about what you look like, even if you are by yourself. Just enjoy the sensations of dancing until you feel as if an invisible, nameless partner is dancing you around the room. Once again, notice your thoughts but don't engage them. Let them drift by. Again, if space is a problem, keep your feet in one spot and let the rest of your body flow.

Dancing with a flesh-and-blood partner is, of course, a romantic dream. The experience of holding and being held, gazing lovingly into the transparent pools of your lover's eyes and floating effortlessly over the dance floor is a pleasure too few of us allow ourselves to enjoy regularly. Most of us do not let ourselves indulge in the pleasures of dancing cheek to cheek with our partner because we think we don't dance well enough. Plus, we think it takes too much effort and expense to get dressed up and find the right club. No more excuses! Buy a CD of luscious waltz music, take off all your clothes, and dance! Play out your deepest Fred Astaire and Ginger Rogers fantasy. Swirl and dip around your living room. Or simply sway together, looking deeply into each other's eyes. No matter how wild or mild your dance, remember to breathe. When you breathe in unison, you will find it much easier to be exactly in step with your partner, which will produce exciting new levels of intimacy and fun.

Buy a CD of luscious waltz music, take off all your clothes, and dance!

THE WAVE

If free-form movement is more your style, you'll love the Wave, a technique I learned from my friend Kutira, who lives in Hawaii and swims with dolphins. Noticing that dolphins—one of nature's most sensual and sexual mammals—moved in a wavelike motion, Kutira adapted that motion for humans. The Wave is an easy, erotic, and effective way to build and circulate sexual energy within your own body and with a lover. The secret to the Wave is loosening your pelvis. Your pelvis is your sexual power center. You need a strong, loose pelvis to thrust, undulate, and swing your hips forward (or backward) to meet your lover's thrust. The prevailing cultural preference for flat-as-a-board abdomens encourages people to walk around with tightly sucked-in bellies. Sucking in your belly cuts off sexual feelings in the pelvis and prevents sexual energy from rising up through your body. It also creates a strain on your lower back. Let's do some simple hip circles to loosen your pelvis and free your sexual energy. Swing your hips in a circle to the right eight times. Keep your knees bent and your feet shoulder distance apart. Now circle to the left eight times. Now pretend you are a belly dancer and move those hips in a figure eight: right, center, left, center. Let it be sexy! Throw in some Kegels for extra juiciness.

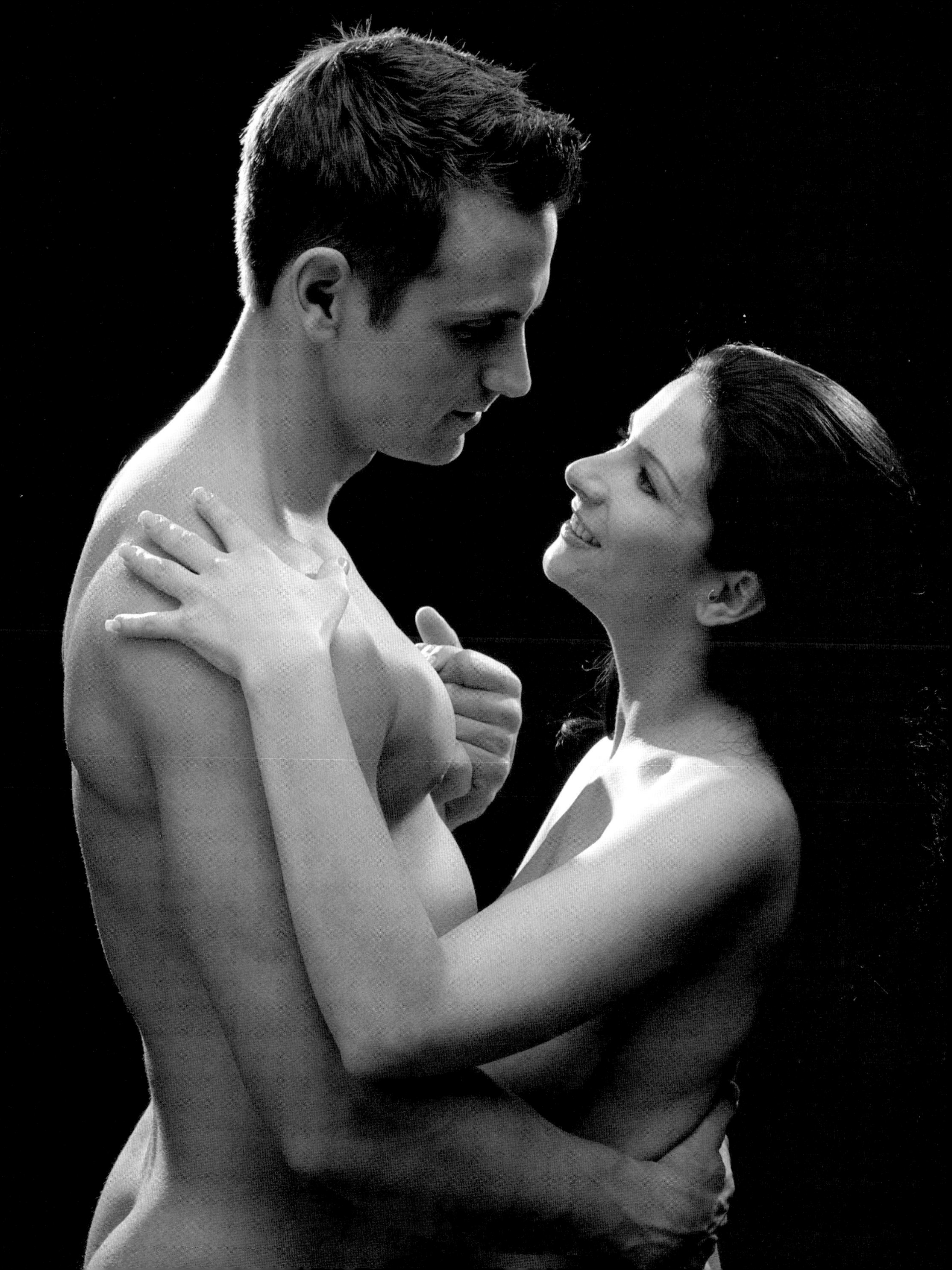

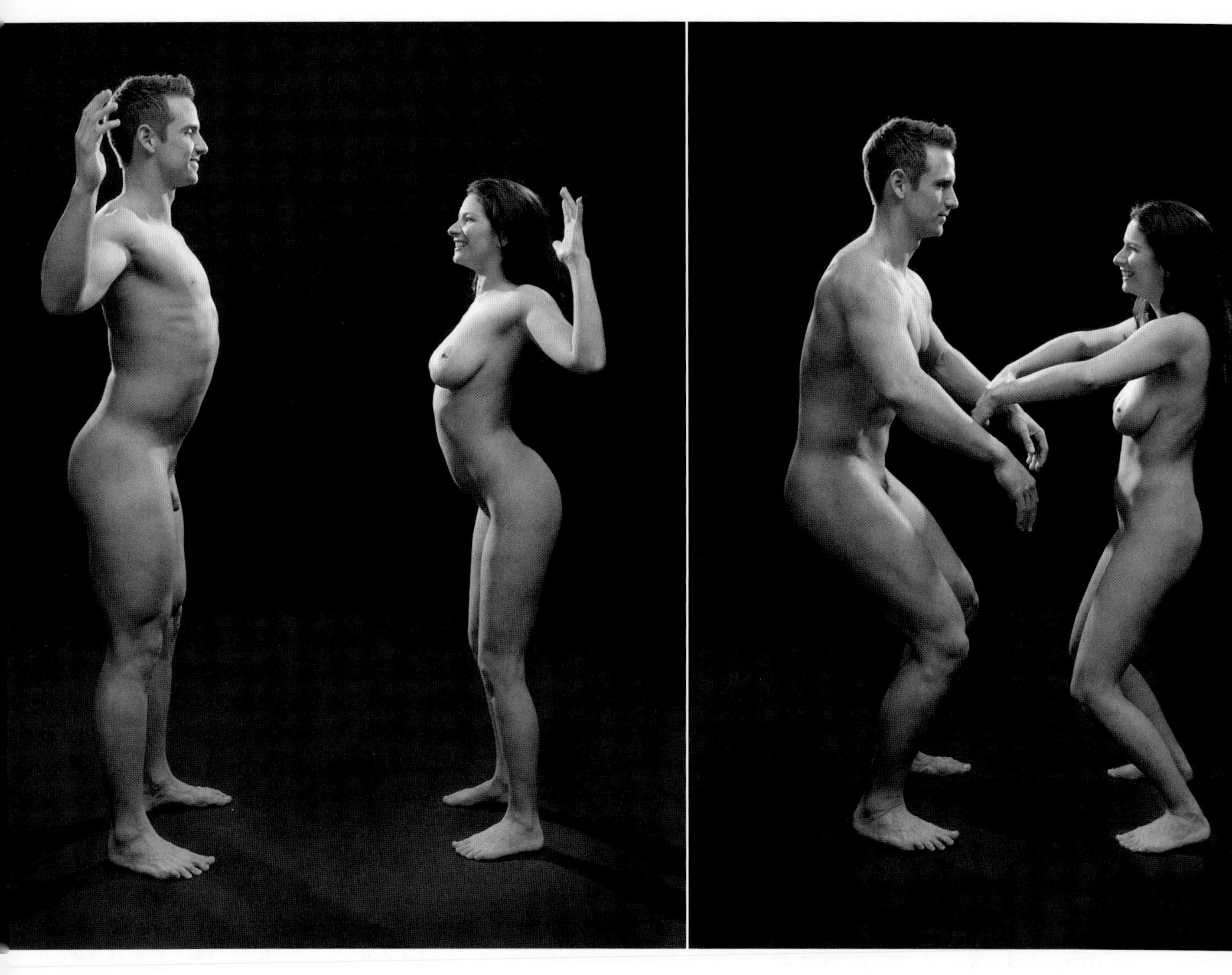

ABOVE The Wave is an easy, erotic, and effective way to build and circulate sexual energy within your own body and with a lover.

Now let's try the Wave:

1. Stand with your feet hip distance apart. Bend your knees slightly. Take a full breath. Imagine you are an ocean wave or a dolphin.
2. Swing your pelvis forward and let the rest of your torso follow.
3. As your breastbone moves forward and up, your back arches. This is the top of the wave.
4. Round your shoulders and your back; your pelvis swings back.
5. Swing your pelvis forward and let the rest of your torso follow. Repeat.

Add the following variations to personalize and eroticize your Wave:

1. Breathe fully and deeply as you undulate. The combination of breath and the Wave can be so powerful that you may even experience little energy orgasms. If that happens, breathe into them and, if you can, allow them to get bigger. You may begin to feel like both the wave and the surfer riding the wave.
2. Add Kegels to your Wave. There is no perfect place in the Wave for a Kegel. Pick the place where it feels the most natural for you.
3. Add a visualization as you undulate, breathe, and Kegel. Imagine that the wave of your own sexual energy has begun in your genitals and is curling up over your back and swooshing down your front.
4. Do the Wave with your partner. As you gaze into each other's eyes, imagine that your wave of sexual energy is washing up over your back and head and crashing down over your partner, enveloping her in your sexual energy. Then imagine that her wave of sexual energy is breaking over you.

HUG

Full-body sexercises such as the Wave build up enormous amounts of sexual energy. As we learned in the Clench and Hold breath orgasm technique (page 25), when you build up a lot of energy and then become very still, the energy swirls around inside you, producing waves of bliss and feelings of expansiveness, connection, and vitality. One delicious way to enjoy stillness with your partner is with a first-class luxury hug. Hugs have not really been given their proper due in the erotic arena. When we think of hugs, we tend to think of comfort, consolation, greetings, and good-byes. Hugs seem a little soft-core when it comes to more intense expressions of sex. This couldn't be farther from the truth.

All hugs given with a loving intention are powerful. Haven't you noticed that after you have received a hug—even a surprise hug from a total stranger—you feel closer to and more trusting of that person? Hugs remind us we share with all human beings the yearning to feel open and safe with each other. Hugs help us know that we *can* be safe in each other's presence. The secret to a truly world-class hug is being able to melt into your partner. Being held is an incredibly intimate experience. Many people feel shy and self-conscious about getting that close to someone else, even a lover. However, the deeper we dive into extended states of arousal, the more we find ourselves in uncharted emotional and psychic waters and the more we need the trusting reassurance that the best hugs can provide.

Set a timer for three minutes. Now walk toward your lover and hug her. Just be natural about it. Simply give and receive a hug. In our culture hugs tend to be the length of a handshake, so you may have to get used to hugging for three minutes. Breathe. Allow the hug to change. Move a bit if you need to get more comfortable.

When the three minutes are up, tell your partner what the hug was like for you. Did you feel uneasy? Uncom-

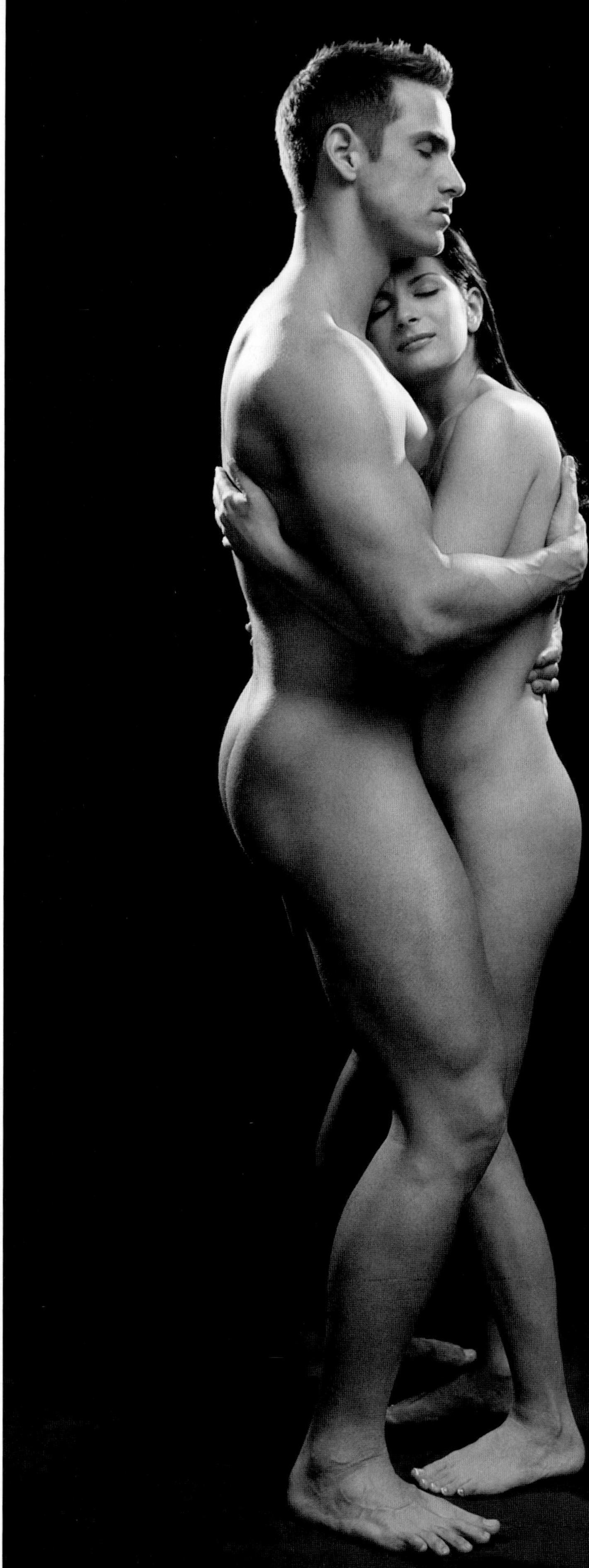

RIGHT The Grounding Hug invites you back into your body.

Hugs remind us we share with all human beings the yearning to feel open and safe with each other.

fortable? Did you like the way your partner was hugging you or did you feel smothered or held at a distance? Did any part of your body remain stiff? When you have finished sharing, listen to how your partner felt about the hug. There is no right or wrong response. Hugging is so simple it is quite profound. It can bring up long-buried feelings of unworthiness or fear. Happily, hugging is also the antidote to these feelings. Two types of hugs that I find particularly intimate and supportive are the Whole-Heart-Whole-Body Hug and the Grounding Hug.

The Whole-Heart-Whole-Body Hug is just that. It's a melting of two hearts and two bodies into a simultaneous holding and loving. Start by gazing into your partner's eyes. Step toward him, allowing your hearts to meet first. As your chests come together, nestle into each other, wrapping your arms around your partner to hold him to you. Relax your pelvis and allow it to come forward until it meets your partner's pelvis. Let your bellies relax into each other. Keeping your knees bent, let your thighs and legs come together. Breathe. With each breath, commit more fully to the hug. There is nothing to do, or prove, or feel. Just be. You will both feel when it is time for the hug to end. Separate gently. End with a kiss.

The Grounding Hug helps the receiving partner feel at home in her body. As our culture has evolved into more of a service economy than a manufacturing economy, the activities of our daily lives emphasize concentration, problem solving, and logistics over physical activity. At the end of a workday, we may not even be aware that we have a body, unless, of course, some part of it hurts. Your body wants to take you to new heights and depths of erotic sensation and pleasure. Often the spirit is willing, but the flesh is numb. The Grounding Hug invites you back into your body.

In the Grounding Hug, one partner gives while the other receives. To give your partner a Grounding Hug, stand with your feet hip distance apart and your knees slightly bent. Breathe deep full breaths, bringing your awareness to your genitals. Imagine that your legs are huge strong tree roots anchoring you deep into the earth.

Now embrace your partner. Place one hand on her lower back, the other on her upper/middle back. Breathe your belly into her belly. As you hug, imagine that you are grounding your partner in the earth, rooting her the way you are rooted.

Continue to breathe together, feeling your partner letting go and relaxing. You'll actually feel your partner's center of gravity move down into her pelvis and legs.

Switch positions; now it's your turn to receive. Receive the Grounding Hug with as much awareness as you gave it.

When you have both received the Grounding Hug, go back into the Whole-Heart-Whole-Body Hug. Let yourself start to move again. Let your pelvis sway back and forth. Grind your hips into your partner's. Let it get sexy. Allow the dance the two of you create together to move you into your next erotic adventure.

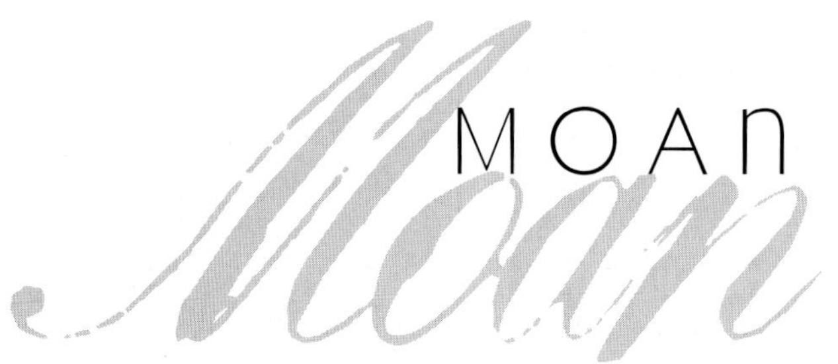

MOAN

WHAT SOUNDS DO YOU THINK of when you are thinking of sex? Intimate conversation? Naughty sex talk? Moans and groans? Oohs and Aahs? Ohmigod, yessss? Crying? Laughing? Screaming? Sounds are an inseparable part of sex. When you close your eyes, you are making love in your own personal erotic soundscape. You may like to whisper your dirty desires into your partner's ear. You may like hearing your lover talk dirty to you. Or you may love the nonverbal sounds of sex: the grunts, gasps, and panting. Or perhaps you like high-volume screams and cries and wails. Whatever your preferences, sound is a hugely important erotic energy gener-ator. You can use sound mindfully to build the erotic charge between you and your partner, even to the extent of having a "soundgasm."

OPPOSITE You can use sound mindfully to build the erotic charge between you and your partner, even to the extent of having a "soundgasm."

6

Release Sound, Release Stress

Sound is not only a great way to raise sexual energy. It's also an effective way to clear out the built-up emotional gunk that we all collect as we walk—or run—through our daily lives. It is hard to be open, intimate, and trusting with your partner if you have brought home any feelings of rage, powerlessness, or revenge about a coworker or a boss. You can use sound to clear out those feelings, leaving you present and receptive to the love and reverence being offered to you by your lover.

Try this exercise: Stand with feet hip distance apart. Do a power yell. The style of your power yell is up to you. It might be a karatelike *Ho!* or a long scream that releases your inner wild man or woman. Let everything you are feeling express itself in one enormous sound. Still feeling you've got more to release? Great! Do it again. And again, if necessary. Now stand still and notice how you feel. Do you still feel the vibration from that big sound? Breathe. Let that energy resonate inside you and let the vibration flow down into your arms and legs, waking up all your sensory nerves.

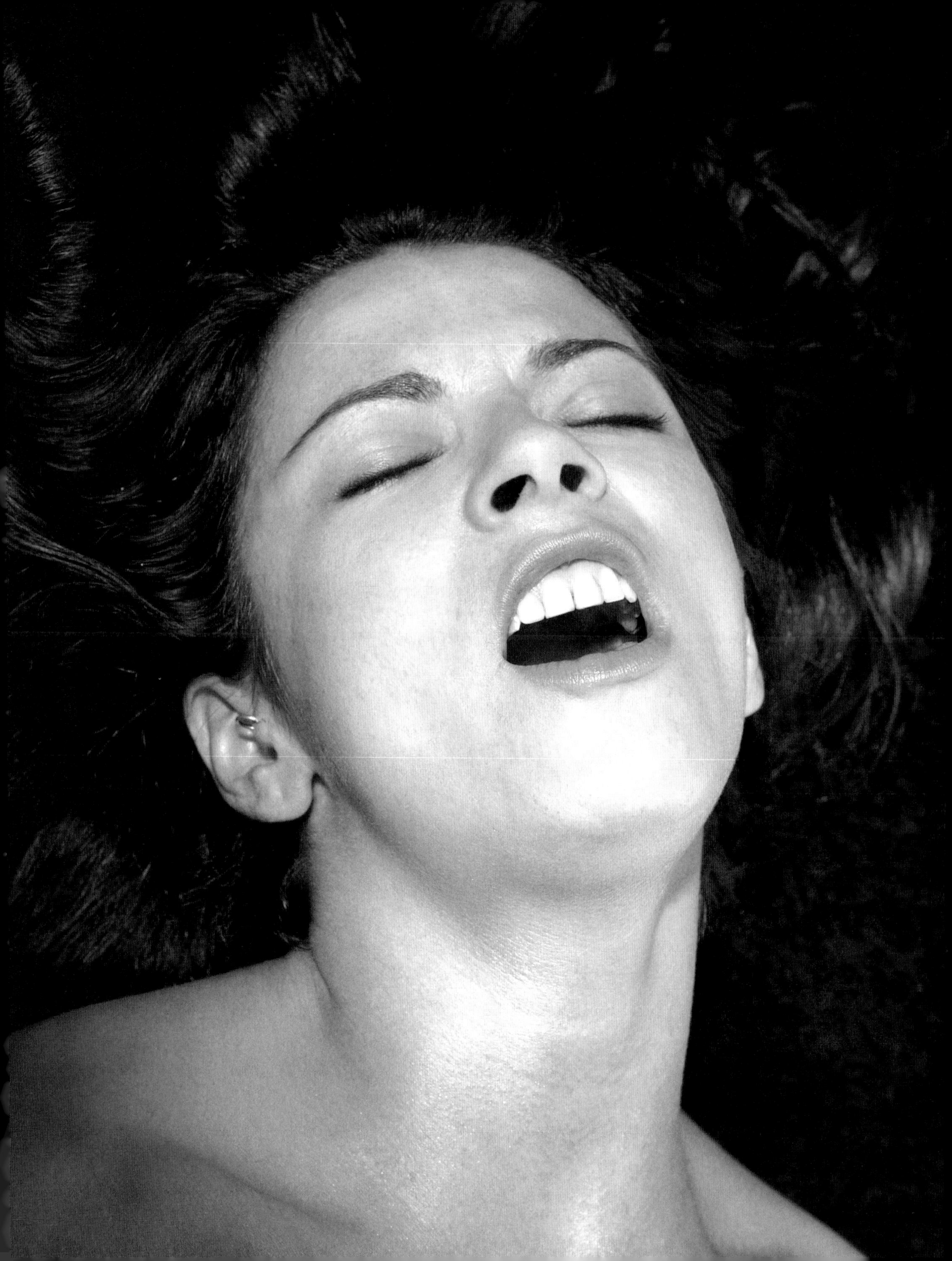

Another powerful sound-release technique is the *Hoo* meditation. Jump up and down shouting "*Hoo! Hoo! Hoo!*" as deeply as possible. Raise your arms and bring them down in time with your exhaled breath as though your fists were sledgehammers. Each time you land on the flats of your feet, let the sound hammer deep into your genitals. Give it all you have. When you are done, stop and notice the difference in the way you are feeling. Do not judge it or dissect it, just notice it.

SEXY SOUND GAMES

If you are feeling overwhelmed by too many tasks or obligations, an even more chaotic technique might be more your style. Explode! Go totally mad, scream, shout, cry, jump, shake, dance, sing, laugh, throw yourself around. Hold nothing back. (A little acting often helps get you started—fake it till you feel it!) Jettison every unpleasant thought and emotion. Keep your whole body moving. Go into it totally. When you are done, you will feel empty and alive, ready to be filled up with pleasure.

If you think that making power sounds in your living room will prompt someone to call 911, fill your bathtub with about six inches (or more) of comfortable warm water. Get into the tub and let the warm water relax you. Lean forward and put your face into the water. Scream. Release all your sadness, frustration, and anger: Yell, "Fuck you! Go fuck yourself! Go to hell!" or your own version of that. Let it all out. Believe it or not, no one outside the bathroom will hear you. Trust me; I have been an apartment dweller my whole life and this technique has been a real life and love saver.

Mad/Sad/Glad/Scared Now you are ready to come together with your partner. Sit across from her. You don't have to sit directly in front. This can be too confronting and too reminiscent of adversarial business meetings. It's usually more sensuous to sit off to your partner's side a bit. Breathe. Do a minute or two of eye gazing. Even though you may have screamed for ten minutes in the bathtub, when you meet your beloved and begin to make love, inevitably new emotions come up. I like to play the Mad/Sad/Glad/Scared game in order to identify and release these feelings. The game is very simple. Each of you completes the following four sentences:

I am mad about . . .

I am sad about . . .

I am glad about . . .

I am scared about . . .

While your partner is telling you what she is mad, sad, glad, and scared about, you say nothing. Simply listen. She will be equally silent and attentive when you are speaking. This is not a discussion or a bitch session; it's an emotional clearing exercise. You will probably discover that whatever is making your partner mad, sad, scared, and even glad has nothing to do with you. Repeat this exercise until you can both move into passion with a feeling of openness, trust, and peace. If anything comes up that might merit further discussion, agree to set it aside to discuss later if it's still on your mind. I find this exercise incredibly freeing. No matter how open and loving I want to be when I approach my partner with the intention of making love, I usually find that I am bringing outside worries into the bedroom. It's inevitable. Sexual intimacy is similar to a powerful meditation in that raising sexual energy brings up all our feelings—the fearful ones as well as the ecstatic. After I play Mad/Sad/Glad/Scared, I feel as if I have packed up those minor worries and put them aside, either permanently or at least until the next day.

Moans and Groans Now it's time to get sexy. One of the most delightful ways to use sound to get your libido rising is to play Moans and Groans. If you have ever seen a porn movie, you may have noticed that in the sex scenes—especially sex scenes involving more than two people—the sex sounds seldom match the lip movements of the actors on the screen. That's because after the movie is edited, the producers hire people to come in and record the "Moans and Groans." My friend Annie Sprinkle, the renowned porn star turned artist/activist, was always in demand for this job, because she could manage to sound like a dozen different women in the throes of orgiastic delight. Now it's your turn to be a porn star. Close your eyes and imagine you have been hired to do the moans and groans for a particularly naughty movie. It's an orgy scene and it's up to you and your partner to record all the sounds for this scene. You will both be doing all the moans and groans for a roomful of writhing men and women. That means you'll both make the low "Oh, yeah, baby, give it to me harder—harder" sounds as well as the midpitched "Oh, yes, yes, yes. Don't stop. Yes. Right there, yes, yes!" sounds and the very high-pitched "Oh, oh, ooo-eeeeee!" sounds. Ready? Go!

Really get into it. Feel the low sounds vibrating in your genitals. Feel the midpitched tones resonating in your chest and around your heart. Imagine that the highest-pitched squeals are coming out of the top of your head.

After two or three minutes, take a deep breath and notice how you feel. You may be laughing hysterically. Or you may be a bit embarrassed. But how does your body feel? Is it tingling anywhere? Are you more aware of your genitals? Are you a little light-headed? The combination of the breath, the sounds, and the sexy words will have released a great deal of sexual energy and endorphins, so much so that you may be experiencing a change in consciousness—hence the lighter-in-the-head feeling. This kind of sound fucking is so powerful that I have had energy orgasms just by breathing and making sex sounds with my partner. Why does this work? According to Tantric practice, you can move sexual energy up and down your body simply by varying the pitch of your sounds. When you were dubbing your porn movie, the low sounds ignited sexual energy in your genitals. The midpitched sounds brought that energy up to your heart, and the high-pitched sounds took that energy to the top of your head. You can use your breath and the pitch of your voice to move sexual energy throughout your body at any time during sex. Of course, you can wait for the sexual energy to move up to your throat and cause you to make sounds, but it's much more fun and far more orgasmic when you consciously use sound as a technique to build sexual energy. As a bonus, making sexual sounds will also turn on your partner.

The Language of Desire

As arousing as nonverbal moans and groans are, the importance of verbal communication before and during sex cannot be overstated. In order to discover the pearls of ecstasy buried deep in the waters of prolonged arousal, we need to be able to communicate honestly and openly with our partner about what we like, what we don't like, what we may or may not be willing to try, and how we are feeling. In order to do that, you and your lover must agree upon a common language of desire. When you want to ask your lover to move his tongue a bit to the right, the results won't be pretty if you use the same words and tone of voice that you'd use to get an employee to work faster. Of course, that can be a very hot and effective language if the game you are playing is domination and submission. The key here is agreeing to a style and manner of communicating that works for the two of you. Many, if not most, sexual upsets between loving partners occur because of unclear or unspoken feelings or desires. Here are a few guidelines to help you create your own language of desire:

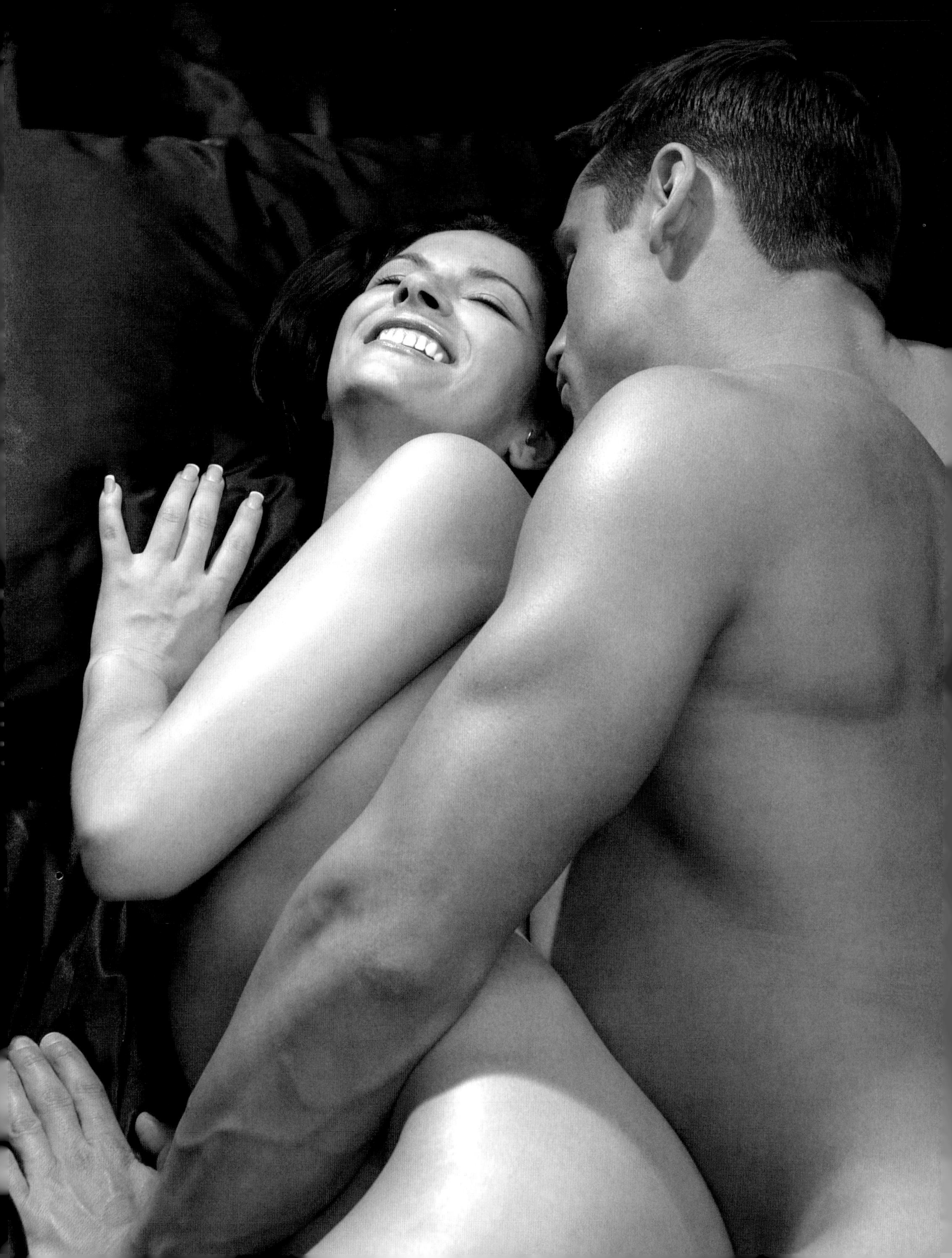

1. Do not try to process everything that is wrong in your relationship before sex. Sex is sex and the relationship is the relationship. Radical as it may sound, keeping some distance between the two is a healthy thing for your sex life. That is why sex with strangers is both an appealing fantasy and a popular reality.
2. Ask for what you want. Your partner wants to please you. Do not assume that asking for what you like will make your partner unhappy, mad, bored, or grossed out. Make an agreement: Either of you can ask for anything you want. If either of you is unable or unwilling to fulfill the request, the other will simply smile and say something along the lines of "Gee, I'd love to, but my bad back won't let me give you that. What else might you like?" Or "That sounds really hot, but I'm not sure I've got enough energy for that tonight. Could we save that for the weekend? Is there something else you'd like even more?" See how this works? It gives your partner an opportunity to give you what you like while giving him a way to communicate his comfort level to you in a manner that won't hurt your feelings or dampen your pleasure. That way you don't have to feel responsible for your partner's happiness and comfort, and both of you end up empowered and excited.
3. Practice receiving feedback without feeling guilty or taking it personally. If your lover asks you to stroke him harder and faster, don't think, "Oh, God, I should have known that; I'm such a lousy lover." Say, "Thank you for asking. I'd love to." This honors your partner for naming his desire and encourages him to give feedback generously. As important, it gives you something to say besides "I'm sorry." Sorry for what? Not being able to read his mind? "Thank you" is much more empowering for both giver and receiver.

Notice how this sort of communication keeps the focus on sensation and on what is happening in the present moment. Remember, your only goal in luxurious loving is to keep your focus on what is happening right now. When you can suck all the juice out of each moment as it comes along, the next moment will be even sweeter.

DIRTY TALK

Some couples enjoy and get turned on by "dirty" sex talk. The magic of using forbidden words is powerful. From a Tantric perspective, telling your partner she is a "filthy slut who deserves a good hard fuck" is as appropriate as telling your partner she is "an ethereal goddess of erotic beauty." The dance of dark and light is a powerful erotic supercharger. How do you feel about talking dirty? If you like dirty talk but are a bit shy until you are deep in the throes of near orgasm, try adding some "naughty" words to the Moans and Groans game earlier in the chapter. Your eyes will be closed and the words will be part of a larger soundscape, so they won't seem so extreme. Once you hear them out loud in all their powerful dirty glory, you may feel a bit more comfortable using them earlier in the arousal stage of lovemaking. Or just pick one word and use it in a rhythmic pattern, such as "Yes. Oh, yeah. Fuck me. Right now, fuck me. Yes, yes, yes. Fuck me. Harder. Oh, yes!"

Some people just don't like to talk much at all during sex. Maybe they are shy. Or perhaps talking distracts them from enjoying the physical sensations of sex. They feel distracted if they have to step into their minds and come up with words. If you are one of those people, you can still enjoy the benefits of the rhythm and vibration of erotic sound without having to worry about coming up with the right words. Invent a new language of sex. Try speaking in a made-up language. Say all the sexy things you would say in English using non-English syllables. This is neither weird nor difficult. It's the sexual version of pet names such as Boo Boo or Pooky, neither of which is English, is it? Your language might sound like chipmunks' chatter or like Teletubbies' babble or like Barry White played at half speed. After a few minutes you'll find that something snaps in your brain and you start speaking and understanding Erotic—your new language. This new language can express all the tender or wild things you might be shy about saying in English. It can even lead to new erotic possibilities. Plus, it inevitably brings humor and laughter into the mix, which builds more erotic heat.

BUILD PASSION WITH LAUGHTER

Laughter has gotten a bad rap when it comes to sex. When people think of sex and laughter, it's usually in the context of being laughed at. We are at our most open, raw, and vulnerable during sex, and many of us have the fear of being laughed at when we are being sexual that is left over from adolescence. In fact, laughter and sex are ideal companions. First of all, let's face it: Sex is funny. The whole sexual act is pretty silly-looking and we would all do well to stop taking ourselves—including our sexual selves—so seriously. Second, laughter frequently occurs quite natur-ally in high states of arousal. Orgasmic energy often tickles our funny bone. When laughter is an accepted part of your lovemaking repertoire, no one becomes nervous or offended if it erupts in the course of lovemaking or orgasm. You may find that winding up in gales of screaminglaughter during prolonged orgasm becomes your favorite kind of orgasm!

Do you suppress laughter during sex? Don't. Right now, give yourself permission to laugh. Genuine passionate laughter builds real erotic heat. When you feel a giggle start, breathe into it. Let it grow. Let the laugh itself feel erotic. If your partner starts to laugh, join him. If you need to, fake it until you feel it, and then let yourselves ride the wave of building laughter together. When the wave finally passes, notice how energized and aroused you both feel. You will have used laughter to arrive at a new erotic plateau from whence you can build new heights of arousal and passion.

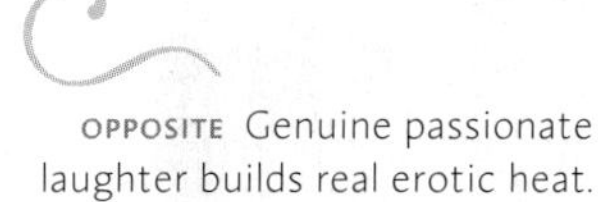

OPPOSITE Genuine passionate laughter builds real erotic heat.

RHYTHM

Last, remember that one of the most primal aspects of sound is rhythm. Everything in life has a rhythm, from your heartbeat to the rain on the roof, to the traffic on the street. Listening to music with the right rhythm and flow will help carry you to level after level of arousal. Create your own sexual soundtrack. Create an erotic playlist and burn a CD or make a tape of music that sends you on a sexual journey. Begin with music (or sounds) that makes you feel relaxed and melty inside. Then pick up the pace with something that gets your hips swaying. Then try a big passionate movie score filled with swelling crescendos. Follow that with hard-driving bang-me-now rock. End with space music or recordings of thunderstorms or raging oceans. Let your sex soundtrack be as corny and obvious as you like. Every movie soundtrack is composed and orchestrated to magnify and intensify the audience's emotionalresponse to the story on the screen. Your sex soundtrack is designed to do the same for your lovemaking.

Sounds are an aphrodisiac whether you are making them or listening to them. If you are still shy about being loud and proud in your sexual passion, practice alone first. Turn on music loud enough to drown out any sounds you will make and start masturbating. Pretend the music is your passionate, loud lover. First let the music turn you on—let it get you hotter and hotter. Now make sounds of your own. Talk back to this loud, hot lover. Tell him what you like and how you like it. Imagine that your throat is a sex organ and that it's the vibration of your voice that is going to make you come. Really go for it! Now let yourself orgasm and enjoy that soundgasm!

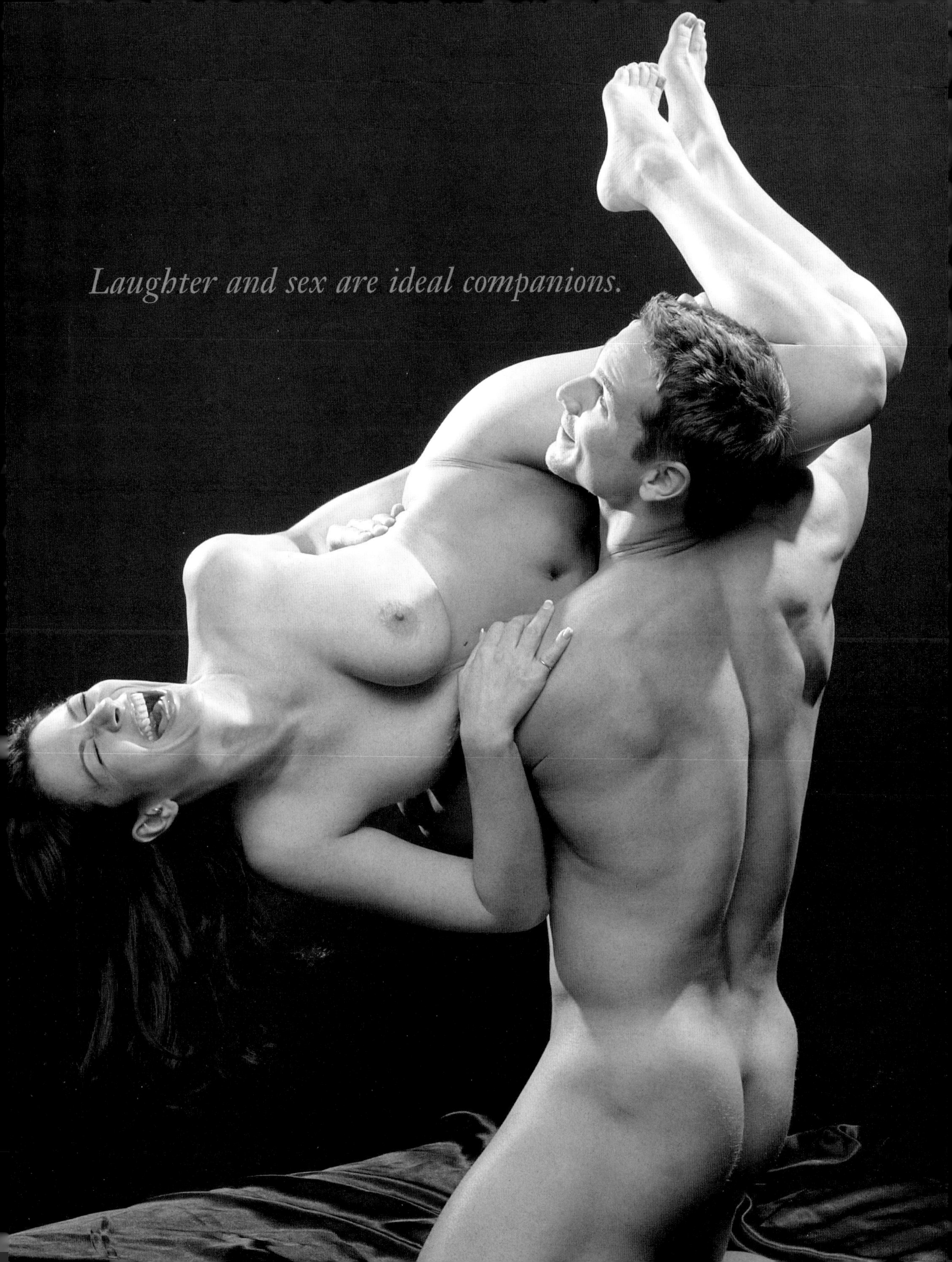
Laughter and sex are ideal companions.

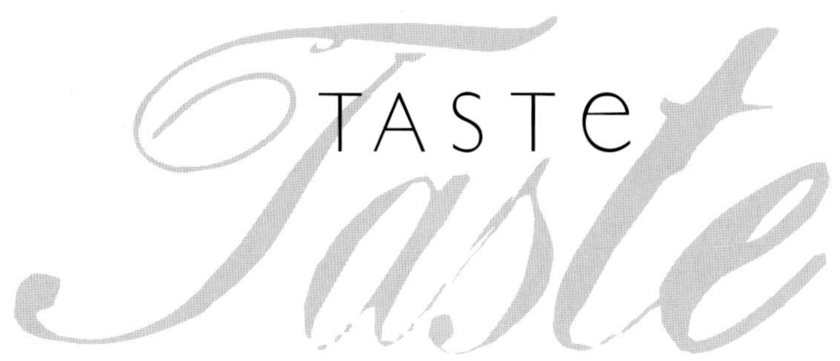

TASTE

7

THE EROTIC POWER OF FOOD HAS has been documented for centuries. Casanova shared oysters with his para mours to whet their sexual appetites. Lovers in both Greek and Roman cultures enjoyed ripe fruits and exotic dishes before engaging in sensuous pleasures. And it has long been said that a delicious meal is the quickest way to a lover's heart. Who hasn't indulged in the sensuous pleasure of a romantic dinner?

What exactly is it about food that sparks the erotic imagination and the libido? Is it the look or the taste of the food? Is it the chemistry of the nutrients and the effect that has on the body and in the brain? Are some foods really aphrodisiacs? An aphrodisiac—the name derives from the Greek goddess of sexual love, Aphrodite—is a substance that arouses sexual desire. In order to be a true aphrodisiac, the substance has to create desire—not improve performance and ability. Viagra, for example, is not an aphrodisiac.

If something were to be a true aphrodisiac, what would it have to do in order to create or even enhance desire? Our sex drive—whatever our gender—is controlled by our hormone levels, specifically, testosterone. When there is sufficient testosterone in our system, a chain reaction will start when we see, hear, feel, think, touch, smell, or otherwise encounter something sexually stimula-ting. Signals are sent from the limbic lobe of the brain via the nervous system to the pelvic region. These signals tell the blood vessels there to dilate, and this dilation creates an erection in both men and women. (In women the erectile tissues are the clitoris and the urethral sponge including the G-spot.) The blood vessels then close so that those erectile tissues stay erect. Erection is accompanied by an increasing heart rate, while at the same time, our brains release neurotransmitters that tell our bodies that this is all good and pleasurable. So what might we ingest to get all that happening?

OPPOSITE You'll be amazed at how much more there is to experience in a single taste.

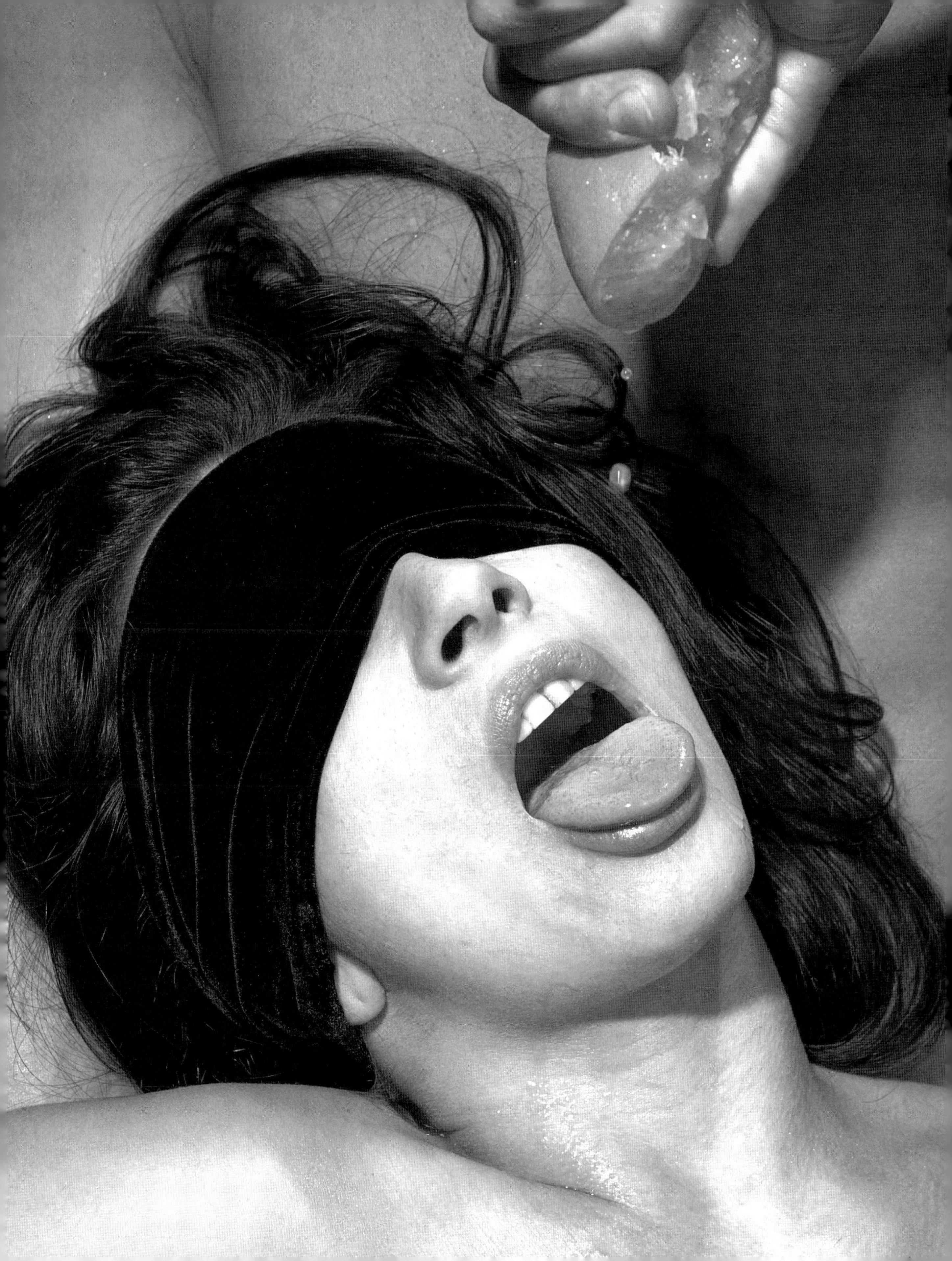

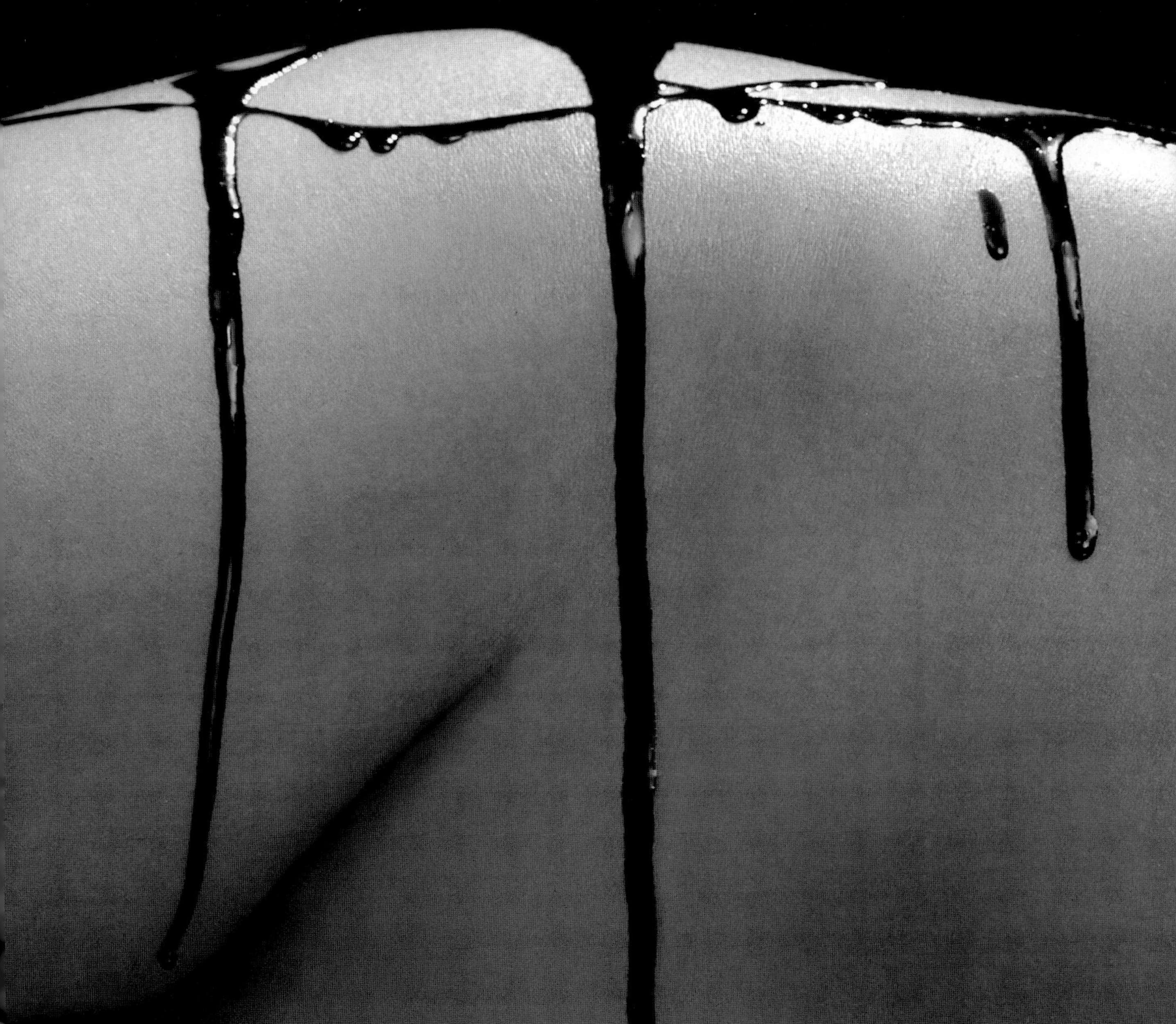

Luxurious Aphrodisiacs

For centuries certain foods have had reputations as aphrodisiacs. Can certain foods really light the brain's erotic fuse? Let's look at some of the most commonly eroticized foods.

OYSTERS

Oysters are one of the oldest documented aphrodisiacs. Although they are high in zinc, which has been associated with improving sexual potency in men, the arousing quality of oysters has largely been thought to be their resemblanceto the female labia. Recently, however, mussels, clams, and oysters have been found to contain compounds that may be effective in releasing sex hormones such as testosterone and estrogen. It has not been determined whether there are enough of those compounds in the shellfish to make any difference. But go ahead, try them for yourself!

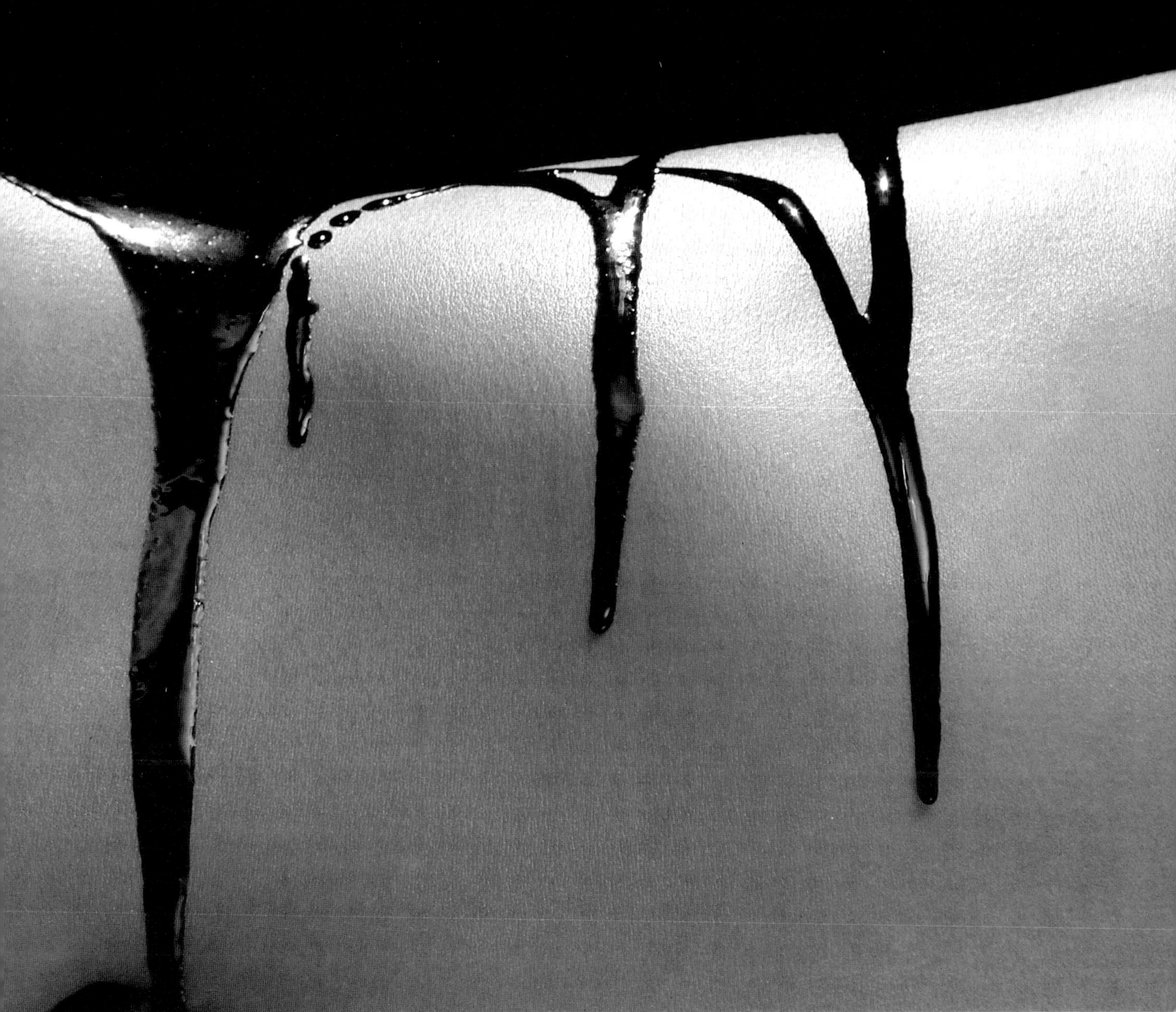

CHOCOLATE

Chocolate has always been associated with love and romance. Originally found in the South American rain forests, the cacao tree was worshiped by Mayan civilizations and called "food of the gods." Legend has it that the Aztec ruler Montezuma drank fifty goblets of chocolate each day to enhance his sexual abilities.

Chocolate contains theobromine, caffeine, phenyle-thylamine and anandamide, all chemicals that are known to affect the brain. Theobromine and caffeine are stimulants. The phenylethylamine combines with dopamine in the brain to produce a mild antidepressant effect, and the anandamide produces feelings of calm and well-being.

Researchers at the Neuroscience Institute in San Diego, California, say that the neurotransmitter anandamide has the same effect on the brain as marijuana. The amount of anandamide in chocolate is not enough to get a person high, but it could be enough to contribute to the mild euphoria chocolate can produce. Of course, this does not necessarily mean that chocolate actually increases sexual desire, but when you feel good you are certainly more likely to be interested in sex. Experiment for yourself.

BANANAS

Bananas have plentiful amounts of potassium and B vitamins, which are said to be necessary for sex-hormone production. However, it is the phallic shape of the banana that is most likely responsible for its amorous reputation.

OTHER VEGETABLES AND NUTS

The supposedly arousing effects of avocados, carrots, cucumbers, and figs are also related to their appearance. The avocado tree was called a "testicle tree" by the Aztecs because its fruit hangs in pairs on the tree, resembling the male testicles. An open fig resembles female sex organs. In addition to its phallic appearance, the scent of cucumber is also believed by some to stimulate women by increasing blood flow to the vagina.

HERBS AND SPICES

Several spices and herbs are known as aphrodisiacs because of their ability to increase blood flow. Cardamom is high in cineole, which can increase blood flow in areas where it is topically applied. The capsaicin in chili peppers produces sweating, increased heart rate, and circulation—all reactions that are similar to those experienced when having sex. Basil's reputation for boosting both the sex drive and fertility is similarly thought to promote circulation. Garlic and ginger also stimulate the circulatory system.

HONEY

Honey has long been associated with sex and fertility. In medieval times, newlyweds would drink mead—a powerfully intoxicating fermented beverage made of honey and water—during the first month of marriage to increase virility and fertility. Thus, the first month of marriage became a honey-moon. Honey is rich in B vitamins, which support testosterone production, as well as boron, which helps the body metabolize and use estrogen. If you want to honey-moon with your lover, you can find recipes for mead on the Internet.

The extensive list of potential aphrodisiacs goes on to include tomatoes, licorice, anise, nutmeg, papaya, pine nuts, shrimp, olives, apples, asparagus, not to mention a host of herbs, potions, and scents. I wouldn't put them all into a blender and hope for passion, but it could be useful to pay attention to the effects certain foods have on your libido.

Some say the power of aphrodisiacs is all in our heads. If we think something is going to put us into the mood for love, it probably will. It is possible, however, that there is some historic basis for the aphrodisiac effects of certain foods. Overall nutrition was certainly not as good centuries ago as it is today. In fact, many people's diets were very poor. Eating something that was rich in nutrients would have had a much more significant positive effect on health, which in turn would have affected sexual desire, making it appear that the food, herb, or supplement had aphrodisiac qualities. People are simply healthier now than in the past, so it's more difficult to see the effects of particular nutrient-rich foods.

In my view, if a particular food tastes good and it's fun to play with, it's arousing. Just the experience of slowing down your eating enough to truly experience all the properties of the food—taste, temperature, texture, and smell—is erotic. However, certain foods will certainly support you in your desire for intense, prolonged arousal, while others will hold you back. The typical big romantic dinner, filled with high-fat food, a sugary dessert, and one too many glasses of wine is a combination guaranteed to produce a great nap, but not much other action in bed. Research has shown that men's testosterone levels plummet within four hours of a high-fat meal. As testosterone is just as important for women's arousal as it is for a man's, we can conclude the same is probably true for her. A much more appropriate meal might be found in a Japanese restaurant. A light meal of fish or shellfish, seasoned with ginger, horseradish, garlic, and pepper and a glass of champagne would be a much more sex-positive choice.

Food and Sex

Aphrodisiac qualities aside, food and sex just naturally go well together. Both can be stimulating, comforting, soothing, nourishing, and fun, and both feed a primal hunger. Using food during the excitement phase of sex can set the flavor of the evening to come. For example, a fun and playful time is virtually assured when you turn yourself or your partner into dessert.

Tit cupcakes, particularly popular for birthday celebrations, are fun, tasty, and easy to make. Simply decorate your breasts as if they were cupcakes. The best frosting for tit cupcakes is the kind that comes in cans—it's stiffer and won't melt as quickly on your warm skin. Add all sorts of cake decorations: gel for writing love messages and drawing swirly patterns, chocolate or rainbow sprinkles, colored sugar, cherries, nuts, and candies. If it is a birthday celebration, add candles. Simply stick small birthday candles in substantial dollops of frosting, light the candles and sing. It's a very sexy alternative to a cake.

CHOCOLATE, STRAWBERRIES, AND WHIPPED CREAM

The most popular foods for sex are without a doubt chocolate, strawberries, and whipped cream. Many people fantasize about being drizzled with chocolate, laden with whipped cream, and decorated with strawberries, then lying back as their lover feasts on them. If you have never tried this because you've been afraid of making a mess, buy a thin plastic painter's drop cloth. Place it on the floor or the bed, then cover it with a white or dark sheet. If the sheet is dark, dribbles of chocolate and strawberry won't show; if it's white, you can bleach it afterward.

Buy the best chocolate sauce you can find—milk or dark, depending on your preference. You'll want the thick kind, not the thin, watery variety. Warm the chocolate a bit—just enough to allow for pouring but not enough to make it too hot to the touch. Drizzle the warm chocolate over your lover's breasts, belly, thighs, and/or scrotum. Add chilled whip cream, then decorate with strawberries. Take your time. The application of each of these temperatures and textures is powerfully arousing. Let your partner enjoy each sensation to its fullest. When you are ready to start enjoying your dessert, once again, go slowly. Don't start feasting on the most sensitive body parts first. Begin by tasting just a bit of the whipped cream with your tongue, so gently that he can barely feel your touch. Tease him—but mindfully. Tickling is generally annoying, not arousing. If you focus on really tasting the chocolate or whipped cream or strawberry, the feeling of your mouth on his skin will probably be delicious, not ticklish. Again, this is an exercise in mindfulness. Eat with the same focused attention that you used to apply the confections to his body.

Try these variations on the whipped-cream, chocolate, and strawberries fantasy:

- Lick whipped cream off your lover's eyebrows and eyelids;
- Make whipped-cream bikinis and eat them off;
- Cover your lover's toes with chocolate and whipped cream and suck it off;
- Have a whipped-cream fight and then enjoy showering it off together;
- Make a pretty pattern on your lover's back, then lick it off very slowly;

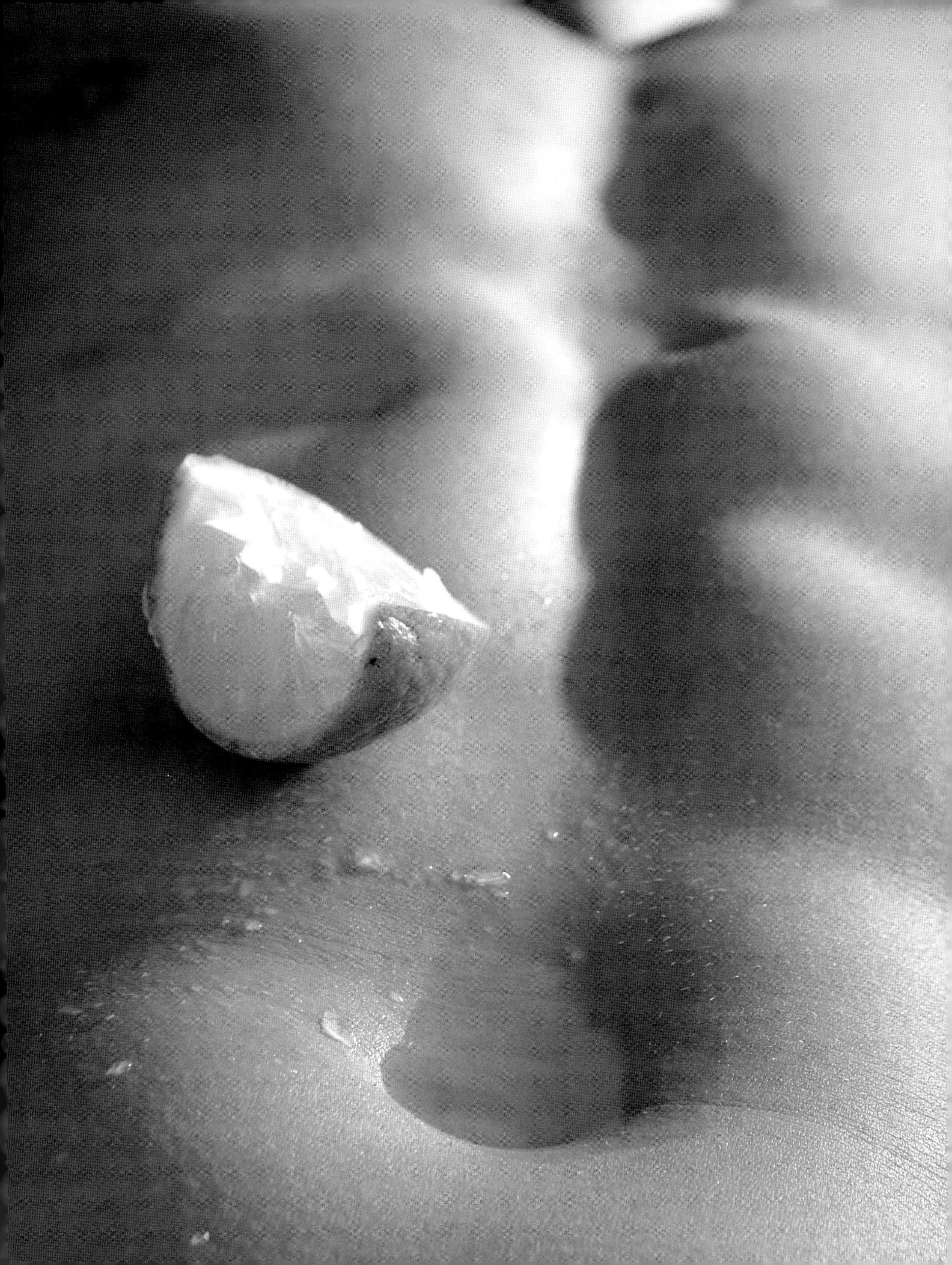

~ Put a little bit of chocolate and whipped cream into your mouth, then give your lover a deep French kiss.

Not everyone likes sweets. In fact, too much sugar makes some people hyperactive, then tired—hardly the qualities of luxurious loving. Instead, enjoy a sensuous, well-balanced meal featuring a variety of foods, flavors, and textures. Include savory, sweet, salty, sour, bitter, and pungent tastes. Spread a blanket or a sheet on the floor and set the scene with candles and flowers, but no silverware. Dim the lights and play music that sets the right mood. Pour a glass of seltzer or champagne. Just be mindful when you drink alcohol. One glass of champagne can be very arousing; three glasses will drain away your sexual energy.

There is only one rule at this picnic: Neither of you can feed yourself with your hands. Each of you will feed the other very, very slowly. Offer your partner just a nibble. Let her experience the texture, the temperature, and all the tastes that can be discovered in each bite. Feed her creatively. Hold a berry in your lips, or arrange caviar hors d'oeuvres so that your partner can eat them off your chest.

Become the Taste

In Tantric practice, we eat as though we could actually become the taste of our food and drink. We try to lose ourselves in the experience of eating, just as we wish to lose ourselves in lovemaking. Food, like breath, is necessary for life. When we breathe consciously and fully, we feel more alive. With food it's not the amount we eat that makes us feel more alive but our consciousness of what we eat and the way we eat it. When we savor each breath of air we take, our breath carries sexual energy throughout our body. When we savor each bite that we eat, we open up all our sensory receptors and we are more able to savor our erotic feelings. In short, the mindful experience of tasting and eating can help us drop deeper into the erotic experience.

Let's try a deeper experience of "becoming" the taste of your food. Blindfold your partner. If she is amenable to the idea, also plug her ears with earplugs and place her hands in soft restraints. The idea is to remove as much sensory stimulation as possible, thereby heightening the senses of smell and taste. Similarly, agree not to speak during this experience. It is perfectly fine if occasionally either or both of you moan, ooh and aah, or giggle. Any nonverbal sounds are just fine. However, talking about the sensations that occur will take both you and your partner away from actually experiencing them.

Make sure your partner is comfortable. Place one hand on her heart and one on her belly. Breathe with her. With your stillness, your touch, and your breath, invite her to relax and just be. You will now offer your partner tastes of a variety of foods. Be creative in your food choices. Pick both simple and complex tastes. Do not pick foods that crumble too easily or are too hard to

When we savor each bite that we eat, we open up all our sensory receptors and we are more able to savor our erotic feelings...the mindful experience of tasting and eating can help us drop deeper into the erotic experience.

chew—choking is seldom erotic! Try to pick at least a couple of unusual items that your partner won't guess on the first sniff, such as tropical fruits, homemade breads, or flavored whipped cream cheese.

Present each morsel differently. Introduce one food by letting her sniff it, the next by running it over her lips, the next by stroking it over the tip of her tongue. Do not let her gobble, bite, or nibble the morsel. For example, a slice of peach can be cool, fuzzy, sweet, and tart. Start by running the peach skin over her cheek. Then place the juicy flesh on her lower lip. As her tongue reaches for it, let her have one little lick, then run it over her lip again and move it away, giving her a moment to integrate what she has just tasted. After you have explored the possibilities of each morsel, allow her to eat it in little, slow bites.

Repeat this exercise with each of your selected foods. Keep in mind that this exercise can be powerfully consciousness-altering. Whenever you enter one sensory realm at the exclusion of others, the mind tends to use the opportunity to travel to distant mystical realms. Your partner may have visions. She may seem to have drifted away. If she seems too far away, touch her gently and breathe deeply near her. Then let her smell a morsel of food with a stimulating scent. Do not break the spell you have woven by trying to force her experience or trying to make something happen.

When I do this exercise, I am almost always surprised and amazed at how much more there is to experience in a single taste. Sometimes I taste so much in one bite that I have memories of a past experience or trip to a foreign land. Sometimes I cannot recognize the taste or smell of a familiar food. Or I may reject the taste of something I usually like. The practice of becoming the taste of the food I eat has taught me how to be more present and discerning in each erotic moment. It has also taught me how to make each moment more erotic by opening my taste buds to the flavors of my lover's skin, genitals, and juices.

OPPOSITE Of all the flavors you could offer your partner, there is nothing more arousing than the taste of you.

OFFER YOURSELF

Offer your partner a taste of yourself as the last morsel in your feeding exercise. Feed your partner a taste of your mouth, nipple, belly, and vulva or penis in the same mindful, slow, teasing way you offered him a bite of fruit or chocolate. Remember, you are not asking your partner to pleasure you. You are offering a taste of yourself as though you were an exotic fruit.

Of all the flavors you could offer your partner, there is nothing more arousing than the taste of you. You may often kiss and lick your partner's body, but have you ever done so with the intention of purely tasting him—of becoming the taste of him? Exchange ten-minute tasting sessions with your lover. For ten minutes, you'll lick, suck, tongue, and taste your partner's body, then he or she will taste you. Before beginning your tasting session, be sure you are not wearing some toxic or evil-tasting body lotion or sunscreen. All-natural body products are preferred. You may want to surprise your lover with a dab of Kama Sutra's Honey Dust edible dusting powder brushed behind your knee or inside your elbow. The smell is enticing, and the flavor subtly sweet. Don't overdo it! The whole point is for your lover to enjoy the taste of you.

If you are the one doing the tasting, start where the flavors are more subtle, such as the ankle or the inside of the wrist. What flavors do you taste? Sweet? Salty? Tangy? As your palate becomes increasingly sensitive, move to areas with more intense flavors such as the armpit, between the breasts, or the inside of the thigh. Save the uniquely complex flavors of the mouth and genitals for last. Remember, your intention is to taste your partner, not to arouse him. When your ten minutes of tasting are up, switch places. It's your turn to become the tasty morsel. *Bon appétit!*

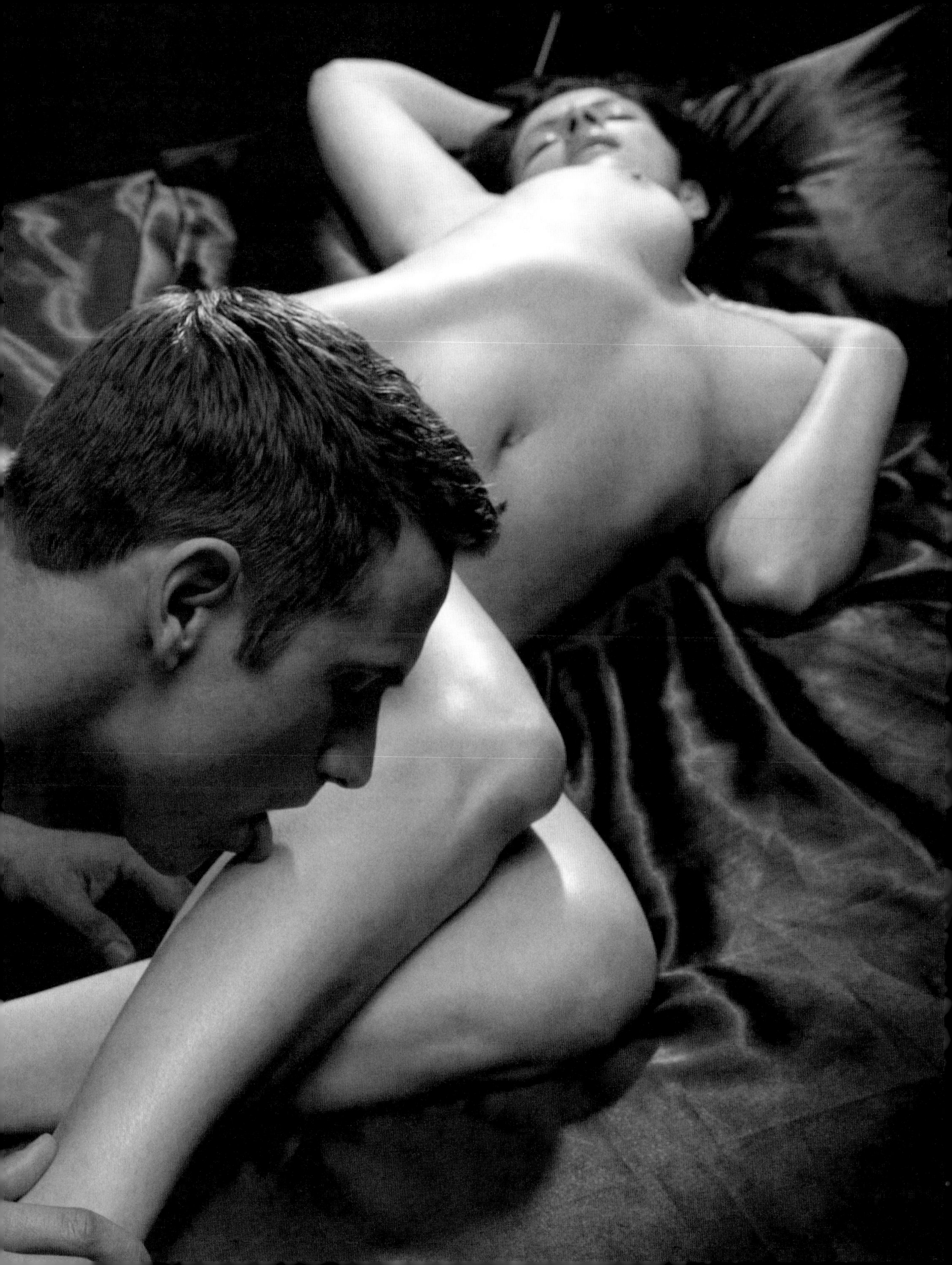

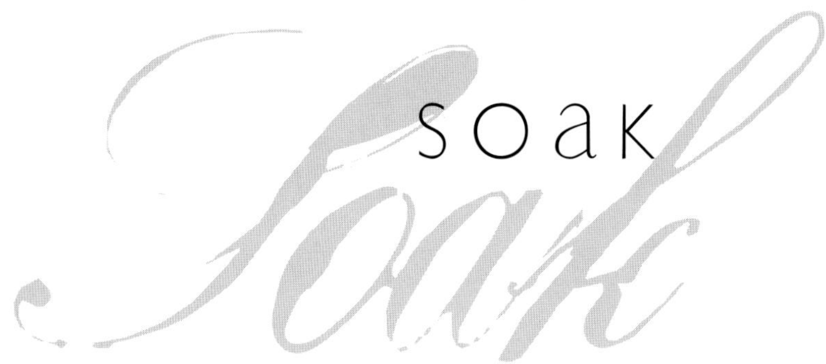

soak

8

I'LL NEVER FORGET MY FIRST VISIT TO a German spa. In Germany the spa tradition is very old and Germans hold "taking the waters" in high regard. The spa I visited was well over a hundred years old and the curative powers of its mineral waters were so legendary that visits there were even covered by German health insurance plans. For me, however, this spa was a water theme park. I had never seen so many ways one could play in water! I was pulled down by a powerful current of warm water into a glistening pool lined with ingeniously placed water jets. After a positively orgasmic interlude in the pulsating pool, I was seduced by the deluge of a warm waterfall that was so completely captivating that a spa attendant finally had to ask me to move on so others could enjoy it. There was hot water, cold water, moving water, misted water, steam, spray, showers, and every kind of hydrotherapy you could imagine. There was a water event for my every mood. Just as one pool of water relaxed me completely, I stepped into another body of water that energized me. Some waters were powerfully sensuous; some made me laugh hysterically. Each new water experience was its own particular kind of nirvana. My day at the spa was one of the most erotic experiences of my life.

We can use water to create states of exhilaration, relaxation, comfort, and passion.

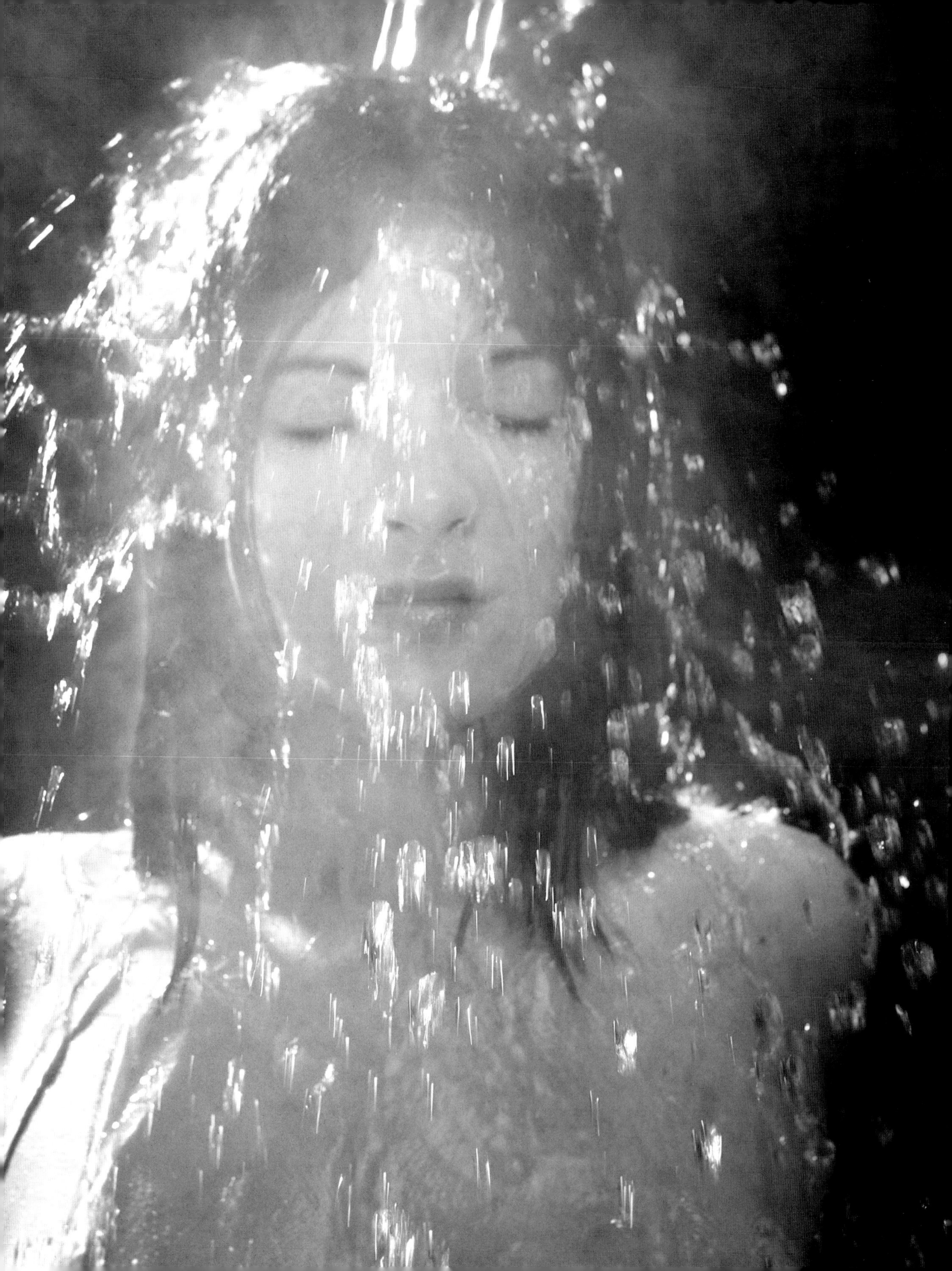

Sensual Bathing

We can use water ecstatically to create states of exhilaration, relaxation, comfort, and passion. Water can enhance every stage of lovemaking and can help you move from one level of arousal to another with ease and elegance. It is no accident that water is one of the central elements in spiritual and religious ceremonies. Although baptism is most readily identified with Christianity, the word *baptism* actually means any water purification ritual. This means that we all baptize ourselves every day. Whether you prefer a bath or a shower, you can give yourself a water ceremony to wash away one part of your day and welcome the next. All it takes to turn a quick, functional shower into a bath-ing ceremony is an adjustment in attitude. Begin by consciously deciding to mark the end of one activity and the beginning of the next with a bath or a shower. Gather your bathing supplies, including a fresh, soft towel, a favorite soap or bath gel, and a loofah sponge or back brush. Adjust the water so that when you step into your bath or shower the water will be perfectly comfortable and you won't have to fiddle with the faucets. Now step into the water. As you do, take a deep breath and let go of whatever you have been doing prior to this moment. As the water washes over you, imagine it cleansing not only your physical body but also the energy field that surrounds your body. Breathe.

Notice any thoughts that pass through your mind. Try not to get lost in thinking through problems that came up earlier in the day or scenarios that might happen later, but do leave your mind open for unanticipated inspirations. As you soap yourself, wash yourself as you would a lover. Then place your awareness in your body as your hands glide over your skin. Now let these perceptions exist at the same time. Feel your entire body relaxing, clearing, and changing as you bathe it. After you have bathed your entire body, wake up your senses by brushing over your skin with the loofah or bath brush. Remember to keep breathing fully. Complete your bathing ritual by lying back in the tub or standing under the streaming shower. Just be. Breathe. Smile. As you step out of the water and wrap yourself in your soft warm towel, delight in your rebirth into the next chapter of your life.

The Essentials

Anything done in water can be a primal and erotic experience. Before birth we all lived in the erotic water world of the womb, in which we floated in the 98-percent water world of our mother's body. When we return to water, we feel our original connection to safety, life, and pleasure. Sensuous bathing ignites and magnifies these feelings. The key ingredients for a sublime sensuous bathing experience are all those you experienced in

Water can enhance every stage of lovemaking and can help you move from one level of arousal to another with ease and elegance.

your solo bathing ritual—water, breath, slowing down, and mindful touch—plus the added essential quality of trust between lovers. Any other bathing accessories are extras, but some are very pleasurable extras that can enhance the mystical back-to-the-womb experience.

Lighting Without question, candles are the ultimate bathing accessory. The way candlelight dances on water is hypnotic. Candlelight also makes wet bodies look absolutely luscious. Get lots of glass-enclosed candles and place them where there's no danger of knocking them over.

Towels Buy the best, softest, biggest towels you can afford. Have more than you need on hand, as getting wrapped in more than one towel when you come out of the bath is truly a luxurious experience of the highest order. For an extra treat, place the towels on a nearby radiator so that they are nice and warm by the time you step out of your bath.

Soaps, Bath Salts, Bath Oils, and Other Assessories There are countless bath products on the market ranging from the purely organic to the completely synthetic. Personally, I am a bathing minimalist. I don't like the feeling of heavy oils or bits of flowers and herbs on my skin and I'm sensitive to too much fragrance. I prefer adding a few drops of essential oils to the bathwater or lighting a stick of incense. I also like natural soaps that offer a pleasing combination of lather, texture, and scent, such as seaweed and oatmeal. However, if thousands of bubbles make you feel like royalty or a box of bath salts drains away your tension, go for it. Just remember that bath accessories are just that —accessories. They are not a substitute for the breath and touch and presence of you and your lover.

Vibrating and Pulsating Water Toys These include waterproof vibrators, pulsating showerheads, and water jets. Home spas have become more and more popular over the years and many home tubs now have water jets previously found only in hot tubs and spas. Vibrating toys and pulsating water are particularly good for clitoral stimulation, but they can also be used on the perineum, the nipples, and the frenulum—the V on the underside of the penis. Remember, however, that these vibrating toys and water jets produce intense stimulation and should be used in moderation when your intention is to build and ride the wave of arousal. Sensuous bathing is unique in its ability to float you away with your beloved; introducing too much stimulation can be counterproductive. Instead, put your pulsating showerhead on a gentle setting and lull your lover into a soothing trance by treating his whole body as a sex organ.

A Luxurious Foot Bath and Massage

Bathing and massaging your lover's feet is an exquisite way of demonstrating your devotion while you help her relax at the end of a long day. Many people love footbaths and foot massages so much they say that receiving one is like getting a full-body massage. Invite your lover to sit in a comfortable chair. Fill a basin with warm water. Remove your lover's shoes and socks and roll up her pants or skirt to above the knee. One by one, gently place her feet in the water. Place your hands on the tops of her feet in the water and breathe. Supporting one foot with both hands, gently lift it out of the water and place it on a towel. While maintaining contact with her foot with at least one of your hands, soap your hands and lather up her foot, working your way up to her calf.

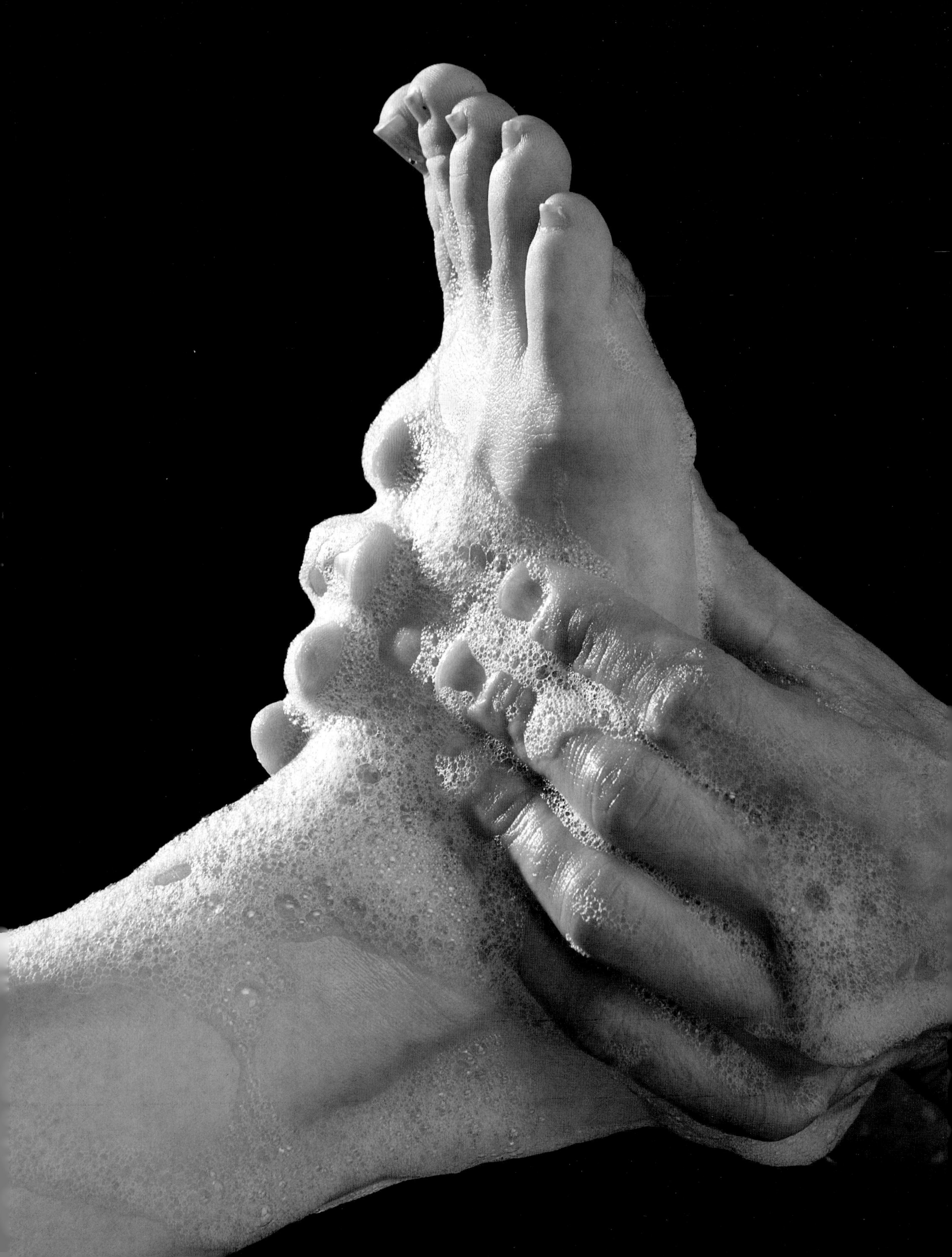

Now place both of your hands around your lover's foot with your fingers on the bottom and your thumbs on the top. Using long, smooth, firm strokes, slide your thumbs between the tendons on the top of the foot from the ankle toward the toes. Work with enough pressure so it's not ticklish, but not so deep that it's painful. Next, massage the sole of her foot. Using your thumbs, make circular motions over the entire surface of the bottom of the foot, moving from the base of the toes toward the heel. Keep the pressure of the circles steady and even. Use a bit more pressure on the heel, where the skin is tougher. Now the toes: Beginning with the big toe and working toward the pinkie, roll each toe between your thumb and forefinger as you slide your fingers up and down the toe, applying gentle pressure. Gently squeeze and pull the end of each toe. Alternate strokes with plenty of immersions into the warm water.

When you are finished with the first foot, gently place it back into the water, supporting it with both of your hands. Rinse off the soap. Now bathe and massage the second foot as you did the first. When you are done, dry each foot with a soft towel and even your breath. Be as precise in your drying as you were in your massaging. Which style of drying fits your lover's mood? A vigorous rub? A firm, comforting holding? A gentle stroking? When both of her feet are dry, gently place your hands on the tops of each foot and wait until your lover is earthbound enough to form words again.

OPPOSITE Demonstrate your devotion by giving your lover a sensuous footbath and massage.

Indulgences for You and Your Partner

Bathing with a lover can be both stimulating and relaxing. Whether you prefer a bubble bath or a sensuous shower, water temperature is important. A warm bath will relax you, but very hot water will drain away your sexual energy, especially if you soak in it for very long. If you enjoy a very hot bath, be sure to follow it with a cooler shower or add some cold water to the bathtub.

MILK BATHS

Naturally, the most practical use for bathing is for cleansing the body. But some baths do more than just clean your skin; they enhance the way your skin feels. It is said that the secret of Cleopatra's beautiful skin was that she soaked in baths of fresh milk. There is actually a scientific basis for this. Milk is a very effective skin cleanser, because thelactic acid it contains is an alpha hydroxy acid—a natural material that dissolves the glue that holds dead skin cells together. But the sensual qualities of a milk bath go far beyond its cosmetic capabilities. Sitting in a milk bath is a luxurious, elegant, and exotic indulgence. Traditional recipes for milk baths suggest adding two to four cups of fresh milk to the bathwater as the tub is filling. I prefer a more theatrical approach. Try pouring a quart or two of warmed milk over your lover's body while he is seated in the bath. Heat the milk on the stove or in a microwave until it's just above body temperature, approximately 100–103°F. Then pour it all over him. The visual effect is as exciting as the way it feels. To make the bath even more stimulating, rub your lover's skin with a washcloth or a loofah sponge. This wakes up the body's ability to feel sensation and also sloughs off dead skin. Rinse his body thoroughly after soaking, but don't use soap—the milk is a natural moisturizer. When you leave a milk bath, your skin feels baby soft and ever so caressable. If you like, you can have a perfumed milk bath. Add just a few drops of your favorite essential oil. Lavender, patchouli, rose, and amber are particularly enticing.

CITRUS BATHS

For those who prefer fruit to milk, citrus showers are invigorating to both body and spirit. Slice oranges, grapefruit, limes, and lemons in halves or quarters and use them as bath sponges. Rub them all over your lover's body. The aroma of the citrus is amplified by the hot water and steam. If you close your eyes, you may think you are standing in a tropical garden in a warm rain. All sorts of erotic possibilities can reveal themselves in a citrus shower. You can suck on the fruit or squeeze it and drip the juice into your lover's mouth. Shampoo his hair with the lemons. Lick the orange juice off his body. Simply rinse off when you are done. His skin and hair will smell delicious and feel squeaky clean.

WATERFALLS

Standing under a waterfall is an exhilarating, consciousness-altering experience. A showerhead, no matter how powerful, simply cannot produce the effect of standing under rushing water. You can create a personal waterfall for your lover at home by simply pouring water over her from two alternating containers. Have her sit in the bathtub. Fill two plastic containers with water. Pour one over her head, then immediately pour from the second container as you refill the first. Try to pour so that there is no separation between one container and the next, producing a continuous waterfall. If your lover needs to breathe or wants to come out of the waterfall, she can move slightly, but the stream of water remains constant. For an espe-cially arousing experience, she might like to use a handheld pulsating showerhead to stimulate her clitoris. Men can use the same technique, aiming the water at the frenulum. This spot is very responsive to vibration. The combination of water rushing over the head during genital stimulation draws sexual energy up the spine and throughout the body.

Create a Bathing Ritual

One of the most intimate times to use water and bathing is following intense sexual activity. When you have built sexual energy to a peak—with or without orgasm—lying in your lover's arms in water will allow you to enjoy the subtlest nuances of the afterglow. A bathing ritual is also a perfect ending to an erotic massage. While your lover is lying on the massage table enjoying the aftershocks of erotic touch, breath, and full-body arousal, you can prepare a bath. Light candles and put on some soothing or inspiring music. Carry (or escort) your lover to a warm, scented bath. Encourage him to keep his eyes closed until you tell him to open them in the darkened, candlelit bathroom. Get into the tub with your lover and hold him. Breathe. You do not need to do anything else. Lying in the warm water in a lover's arms is like returning to the womb; it promotes powerful feelings of trust and safety. Depending on your mood, this bathing session can be either the perfect finish to lovemaking or the start of another round of erotic connection.

Treat yourself to sensuous water adventures outside your home. Unless you are blessed with an unusually large bathroom and an equally large tub, one of the most profound water experiences—floating—is available only in larger bodies of water. Floating on your back with your eyes closed and your ears underwater is like

OPPOSITE The citrus shower: If you close your eyes, you may think you are standing in a tropical garden in a warm rain.

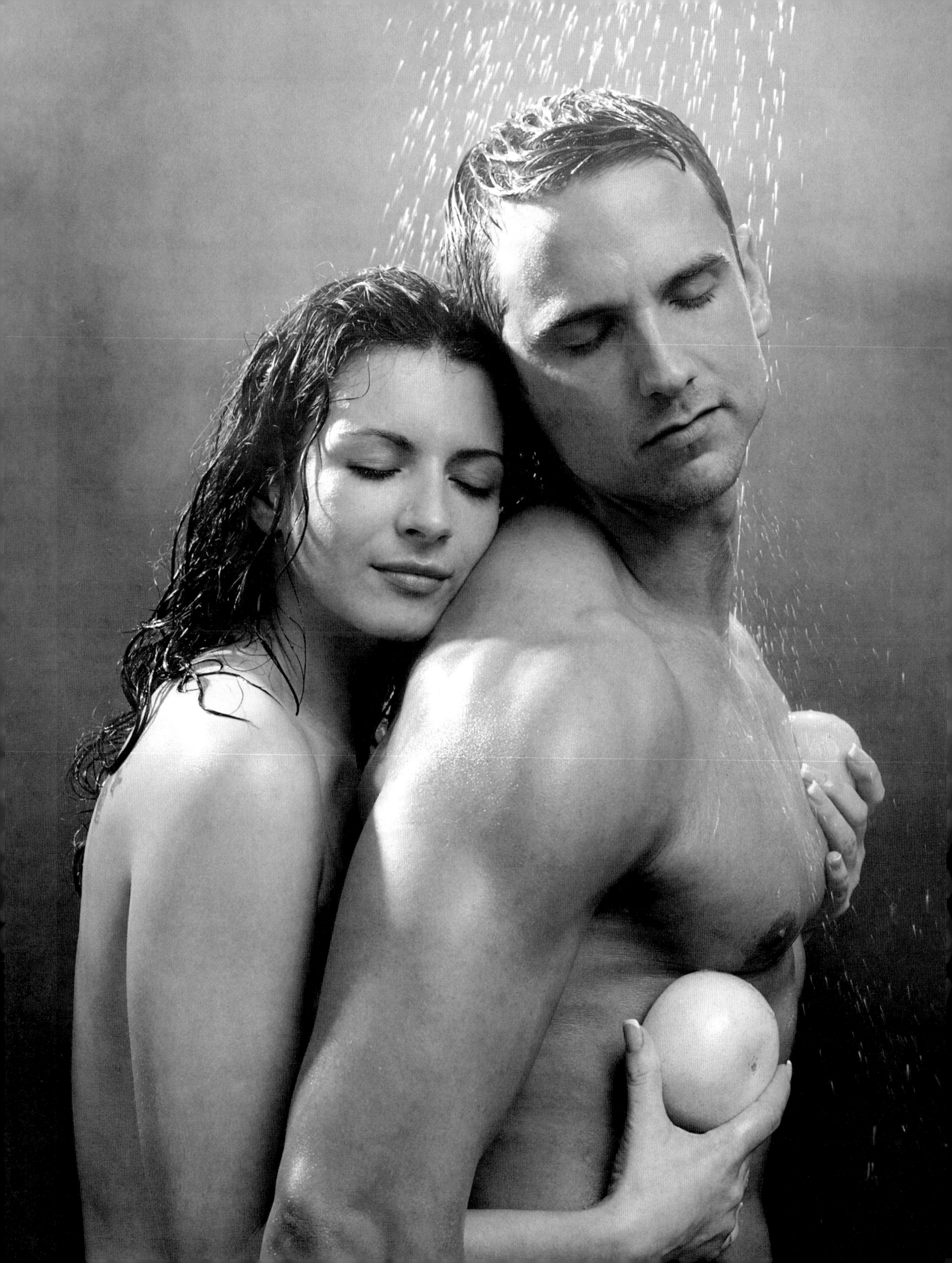

entering a new dimension, especially if your floating is being supported by the gentle touch of your lover's hand at the base of your spine. In this almost weightless world, you can drift into a profound quiet ecstasy. Ask your lover to gently and slowly pull you along by your big toe. He can slowly glide you in circles or spirals, or in any direction that feels sensuous. You can also enjoy wet sensuous or sexual encounters in pools, hot tubs, waterfalls, hot springs, ponds, lakes, streams, rivers, oceans, bays, or out on the grass on a rainy night. If you wish to be explicitly sexual, scope out possible locations during the day and return after the sun goes down, when you are less likely to be noticed and disturbed. If indoor water erotic adventures are more your cup of tea, spend a night at a hotel or spa with a luxuriously appointed bathroom. Pack candles, your favorite bath and sex accessories, and have a long, love-soaked night.

Floating on your back with your eyes closed and your ears underwater is like entering a new dimension… In this almost weightless world, you can drift into a profound quiet ecstasy.

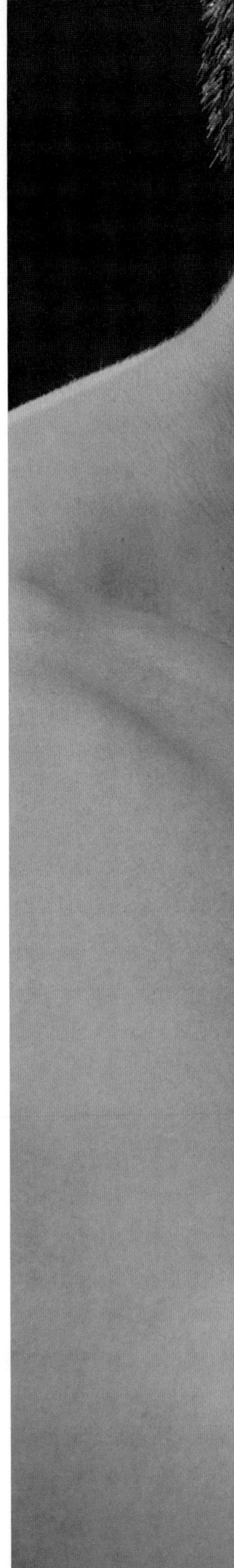

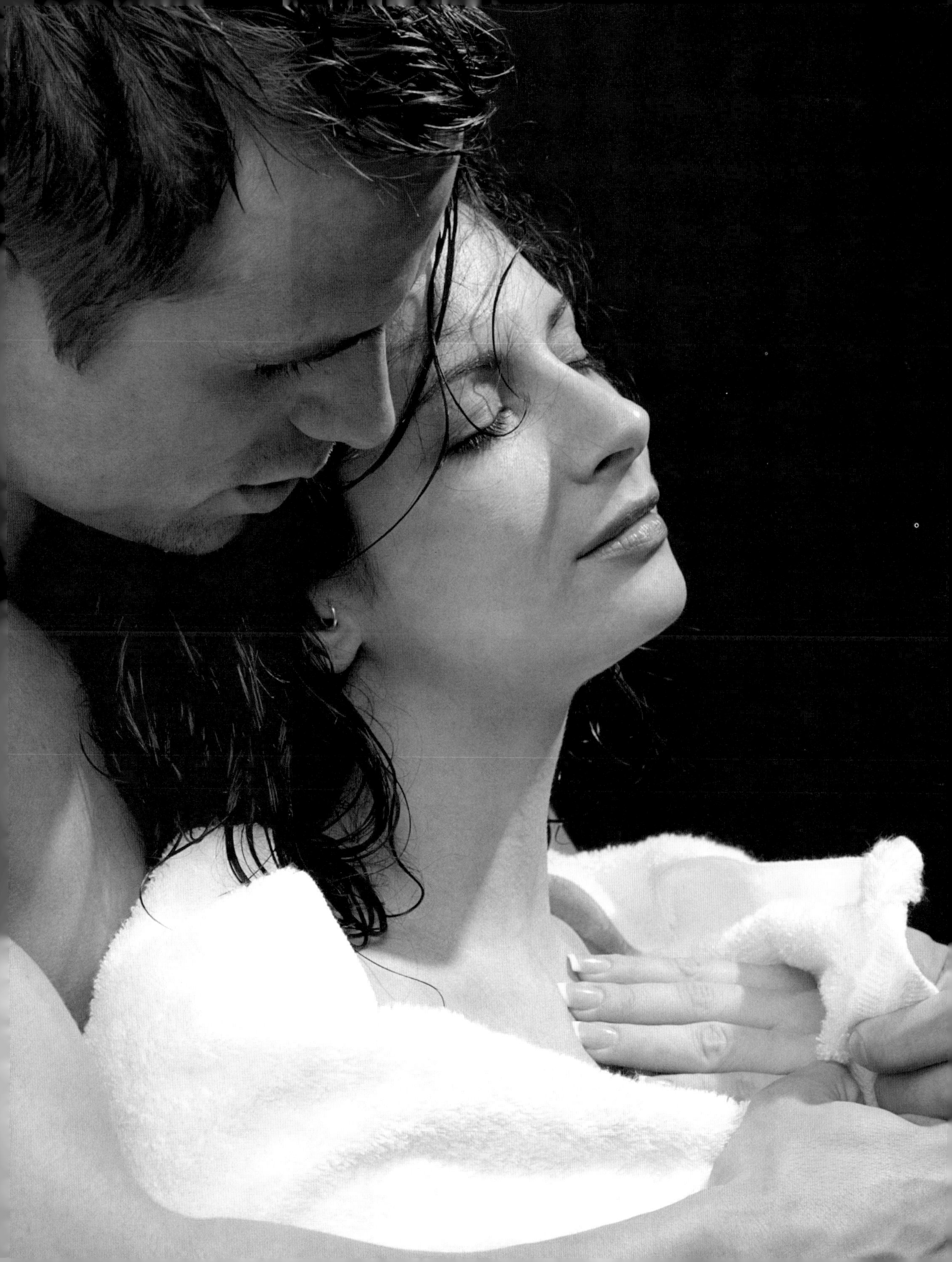

9 Caress

WE ALL LONG FOR THE KIND of caress that makes a warm ball of yum drop into our lower belly and melt in our genitals. Unfortunately, that kind of caress happens unpredictably and all too rarely. No one learns how to touch in school. We all learn through trial and error and by the example of those who touched us as we were growing up. Sad to say, many of us were raised by people who also lacked touching skills. To make matters worse, our culture deemphasizes conscious, loving, sensuous touch and focuses instead on genital, sexual touch. As such we are often unaware of the erotic potential of the largest sensory organs in our body: our skin and muscles.

Our twenty square feet of skin contains forty-five miles of nerves. Muscle tissue and all the connective tissues, such as tendons, ligaments, and fascia, are also full of nerve endings. All these nerve endings produce sensation—a lot of sensation. These nerve endings detect pressure, temperature, texture, movement, stretches, contractions, and much more. All together, about half of all sensory information sent to the spinal cord and brain comes from these nerves. In short, your skin and muscles are like one huge sex organ. The secret to stimulating them is in how and where you touch, which we will explore now by learning how to give a muscle-melting, soul-soothing, consciousness-altering, sensuous massage. Sensuous massage is uniquely luxurious because the person receiving the massage has to do nothing but receive pleasure, while the giver can lose himself or herself completely in giving pleasure. When you can go completely into the experience of either giving or receiving, time ceases, trust increases, intimacy deepens, and you reprogram the way you touch and how you receive touch. The new touch becomes part of your "muscle memory" and you are abler to give and receive exquisite touch during all phases and forms of lovemaking.

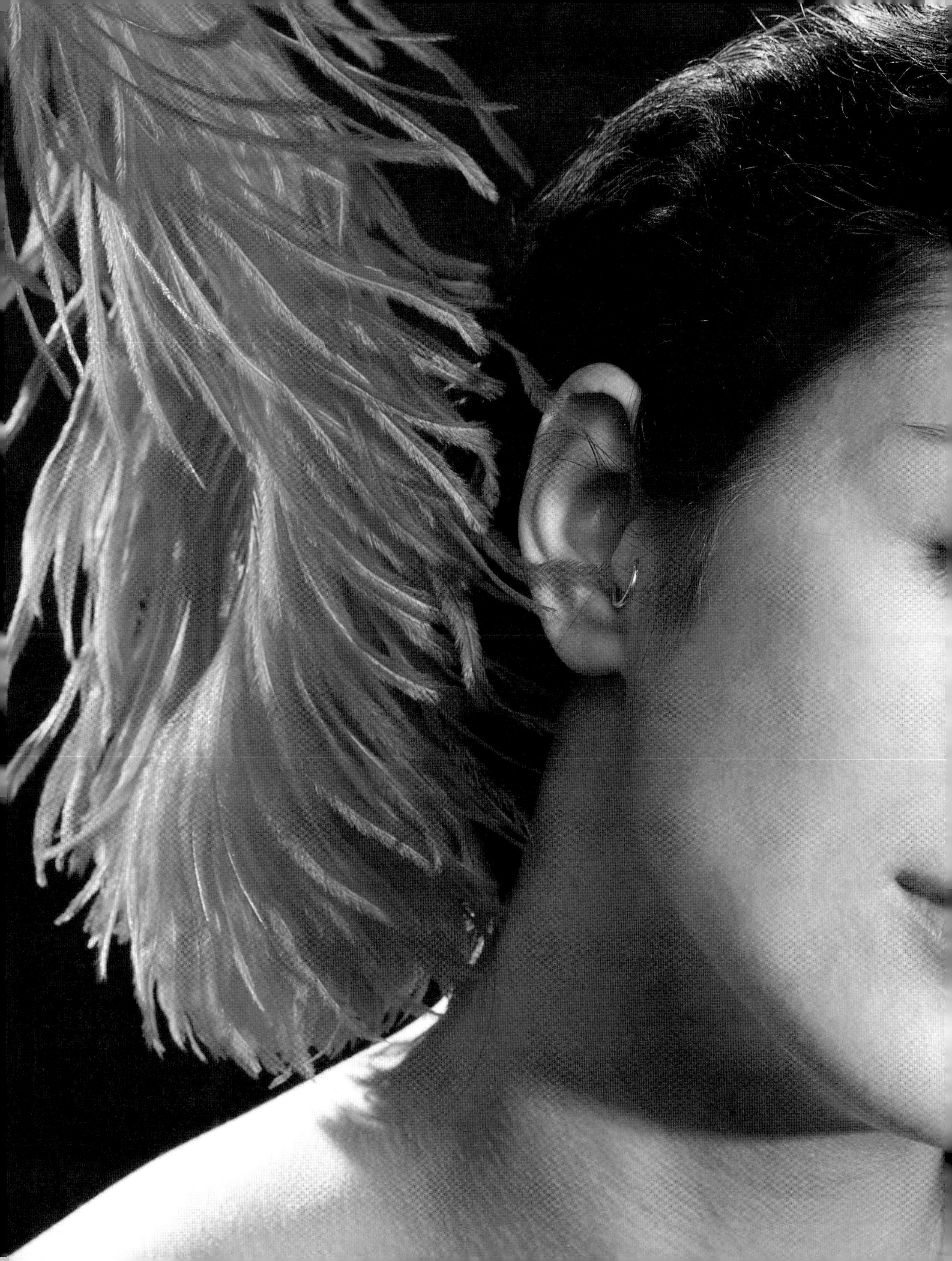

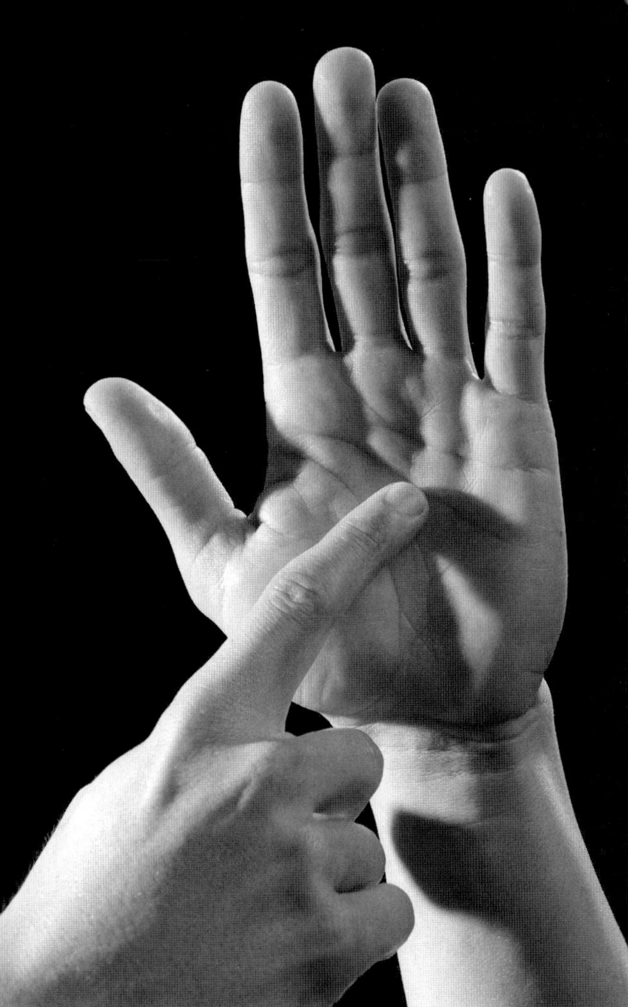

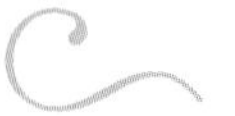

LEFT The heart of the palm.

OPPOSITE Make contact with the heart of the palm first... then let the rest of your hand relax around her arm.

Begin with Whole-Hand Touching

The secret to the magic and ease of a luxuriously sensuous massage is whole-hand touching. If you have ever felt less than competent when giving a massage, whole-hand touching will transform your confidence as well as your touch. When we feel a lack of confidence in the quality of our touch, we tend to touch tentatively. That tentative touch is usually centered in our fingertips and can feel more like a poking than a caress. To improve the quality of our touch, we simply need to shift our focus from our fingertips to our palm.

Find the little indentation in the middle of your palm. That's the heart of your palm. Now touch your thigh or arm, making contact with the heart of the palm first, then letting the rest of your hand relax around it. That's whole-hand touching. When you touch with your whole hand, the receiver feels the touch as an embrace, as if the touch were actually coming straight from your heart. Whole-hand touching also provides the giver with a nice bonus: Your hands receive a massage as you give a massage.

THE FIVE SIMPLE STROKES OF SENSUAL MASSAGE

You'll need only five simple strokes to give a sensuous massage. They are: gliding, kneading, vibrating, lifting and holding, and stillness.

Gliding The first stroke you'll do with whole-hand touching is called gliding. Try it on your own body first, so that you'll learn how it will feel to your lover. Place your hands on your lower leg, hearts of palms first. Let the fingers just relax around the curves of your leg. Allow your hands to conform to the contours of your ankle and calf. Then slowly pull your hands toward you, allowing your fingers to trail behind. Follow the shapes of the muscles and bones beneath the skin. When you are massaging someone else, you can glide from your partner's shoulder all the way down her back, over her buttocks, down her leg to her foot and back again with one long gliding stroke. Don't lift your hands. Go s-l-o-w-l-y. I have never heard anyone complain that a massage was done too slowly. The secret to gliding is to keep your hands relaxed and to pull them toward you, not push them away from you.

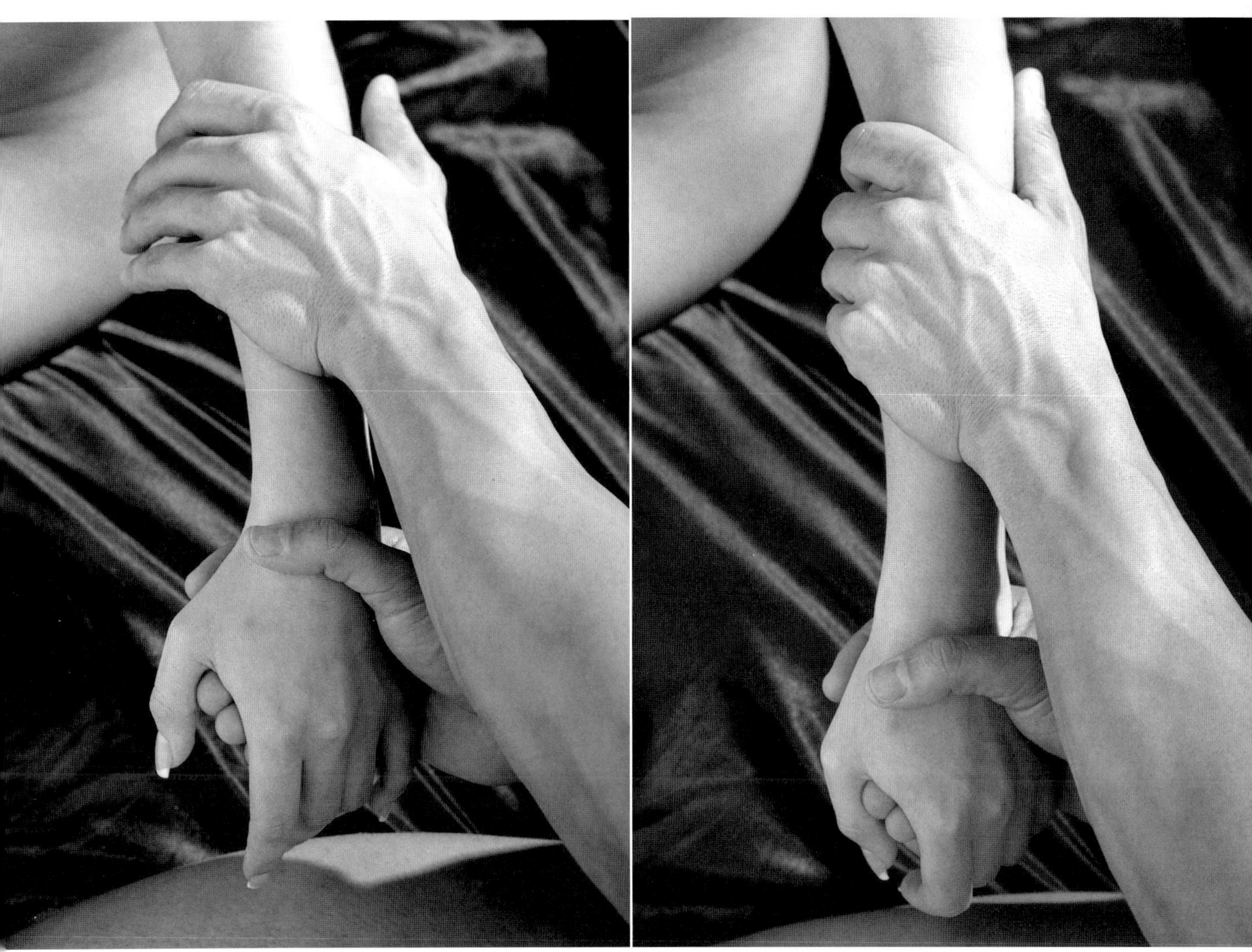

Kneading is a great complementary stroke to use with gliding. Using your whole hand, press into the muscle, then suck the flesh into your palm, the way a kitten would knead its mother's belly to get the milk to flow. Knead with your palm; let your fingers follow. This stroke can feel embracing and relaxing or deep and stimulating, depending on your intention.

Vibrations are a great way to get muscles to relax. Try some on your thigh. Place your hands, palm first, on either side of your thigh. Let your fingers relax. With alternating side-to-side motions of your hands, begin a rather fast vibration of your thigh muscles. Feel the resilience in the muscles and the skin. Adjust the speed of your vibrations until you feel a wavelike motion in the muscles of your thigh. If a muscle is tense, it will take faster vibrations to make that wave. As the muscle relaxes, you can slow down. Ideally, you want to use a vibration that's as effortless and as slow as possible. Vibrations feel particularly great on the buttocks. Vibrate both cheeks in sync with each other, then out of sync, then in sync again. It feels great and usually produces just the right amount of silliness and laughter.

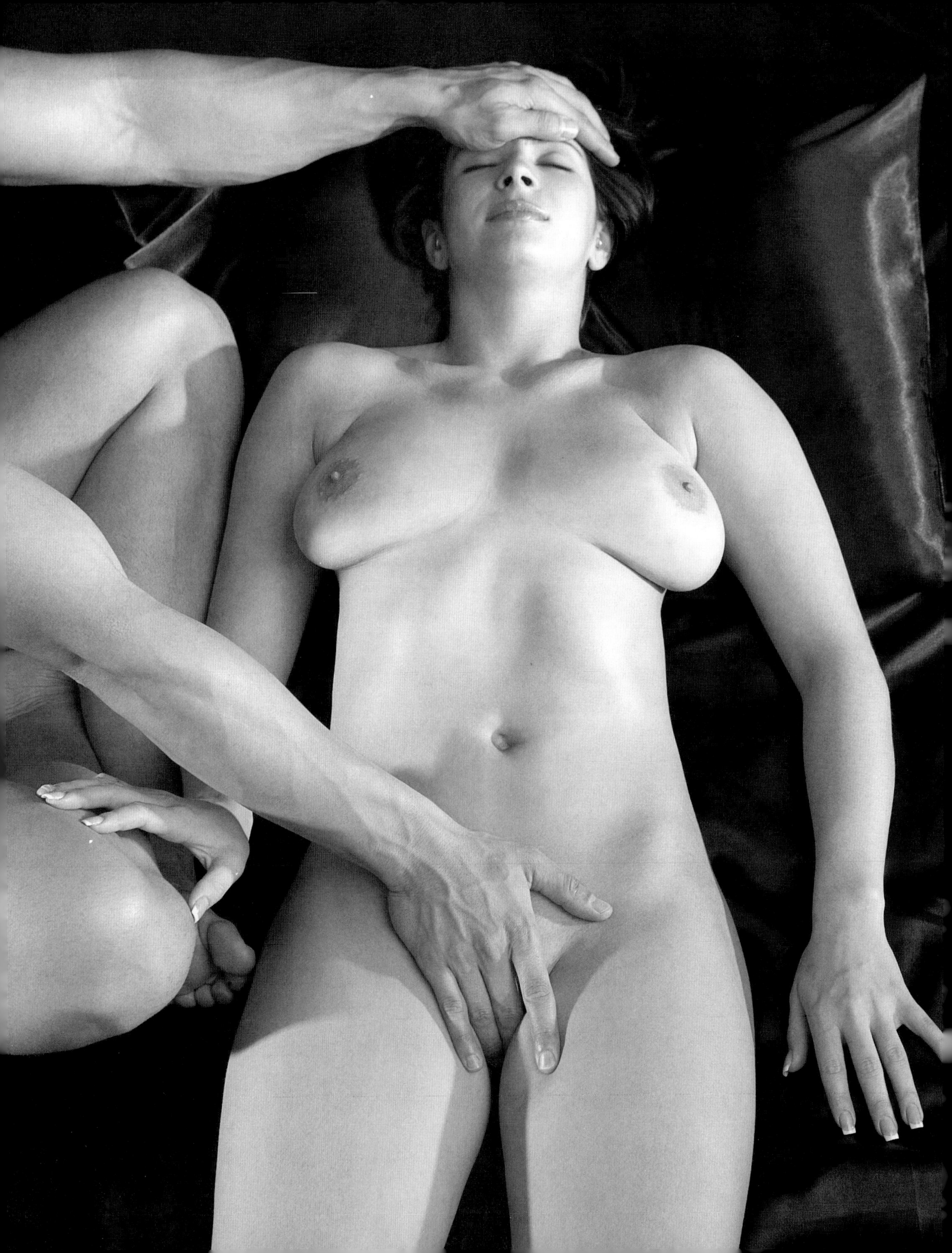

Lifting and Holding an arm or a leg can be an exquisite way to release tension and practice trust. When you want to move an arm or a leg, be sure to support the joints, holding them with the same whole-hand touch you've been using for the other strokes. You can gently pull a limb away from the body and then replace it. When done properly, this stroke is particularly useful in helping your partner relax and drop into his or her body.

Stillness The one stroke that is all too often ignored in all types of massage is stillness. Your hands do not need to be in constant motion. In fact, one of the most sensuous and powerful ways of connecting with someone is to simply breathe in rhythm with her and hold your hands on her body. Stay present—don't trance out. Embrace her with the hearts of your palms. I begin and end every massage with stillness. I also use it liberally throughout the massage to help my partner integrate the touch he is receiving and go deeper into pleasure.

These basic strokes can be used in any combination and on any part of the body, including the genitals. For example, you could glide your hands over your lover's penis, then vibrate your hands back and forth on either side of it, then hold your hands perfectly still as you keep him just this side of orgasm. Glides are also lovely strokes for the labia and could be followed by vibrations on the G-spot. Wherever you are using the five basic strokes, here's an essential tip on how to apply them: Find the resilient edge of resistance. The resilient edge of resistance is a precise name for a very simple concept of touch. That is, when you touch the body, you want to touch it deeply enough that it pushes back just a little. If a muscle becomes rigid under your touch, you've gone too far. If the muscle feels flaccid, you haven't gone far enough. Play with the elasticity of the flesh and find that edge where there is both resistance and resilience. That's where your touch will be the most pleasurable. You can practice the resilient edge of resistance by giving yourself or your partner a hand massage. Or practice on someone who can really appreciate the technique: a cat. If the cat purrs for more, you've found its resilient edge of resistance. If it scoots, you missed it! The resilient edge of resistance is applicable not only to a single stroke or touch. It can apply to an entire sensuous massage or an entire evening of lovemaking. For example, a sensuous massage should not be so soft that it tickles your partner or puts him to sleep. Nor should it be so hard that he tenses up under the intrusion of your touch. When you consistently stay at your partner's resilient edge of resistance, he stays in a pleasurable state of relaxed aliveness, ready for and appreciative of each new sensation.

The Erogenous Zones

Now that we have practiced how to touch, let's look at where to touch. You can give a lovely sensuous massage with nothing more than the five strokes you just learned. They will take you all over your lover's body in infinitely pleasurable combinations. However, in order to move from the sensuous to the erotic, you'll want to stimulate specific points on the body. These points are commonly referred to as erogenous zones. None of these zones will surprise you—you probably have discovered all of them. However, our goal is not just to stimulate these zones but to do so with the intention of building intense, prolonged arousal. Remember, when you are intensely aroused, your consciousness changes. Your biochemistry changes. You become all sensation. You dissolve into pleasure and peace. In order to build this kind of arousal, you'll stimulate the erogenous zones in a particular order.

There are three levels of erogenous zones: primary, secondary, and tertiary.

a

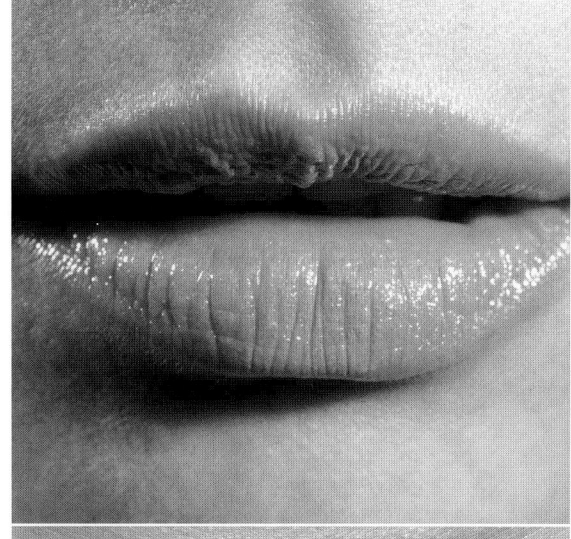

b

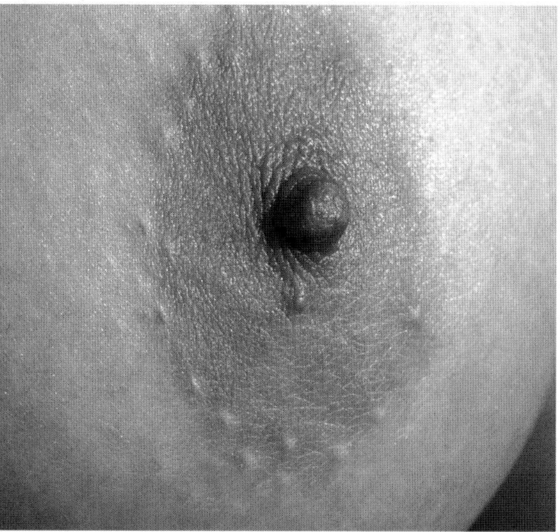

c

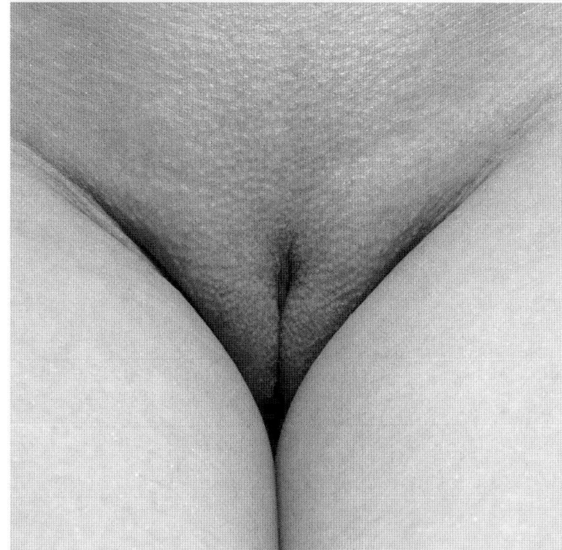

The Primary Erogenous Zones

The primary zones are:

a The mouth,
b The breast and nipples,
c The genitals.

When you go completely into the experience of either giving or receiving, time ceases, trust increases, intimacy deepens, and you reprogram the way you touch and how you receive touch.

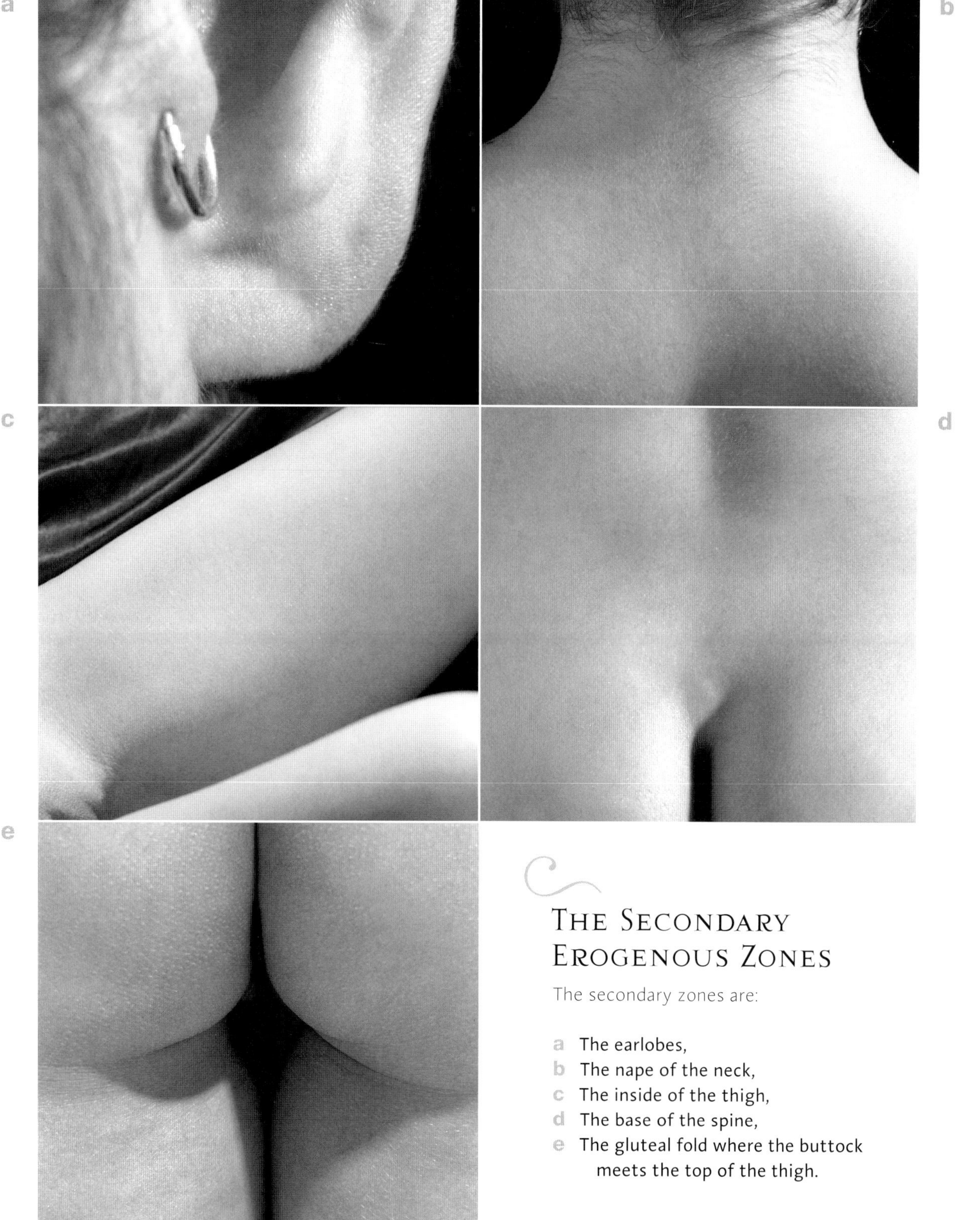

The Secondary Erogenous Zones

The secondary zones are:

a The earlobes,
b The nape of the neck,
c The inside of the thigh,
d The base of the spine,
e The gluteal fold where the buttock meets the top of the thigh.

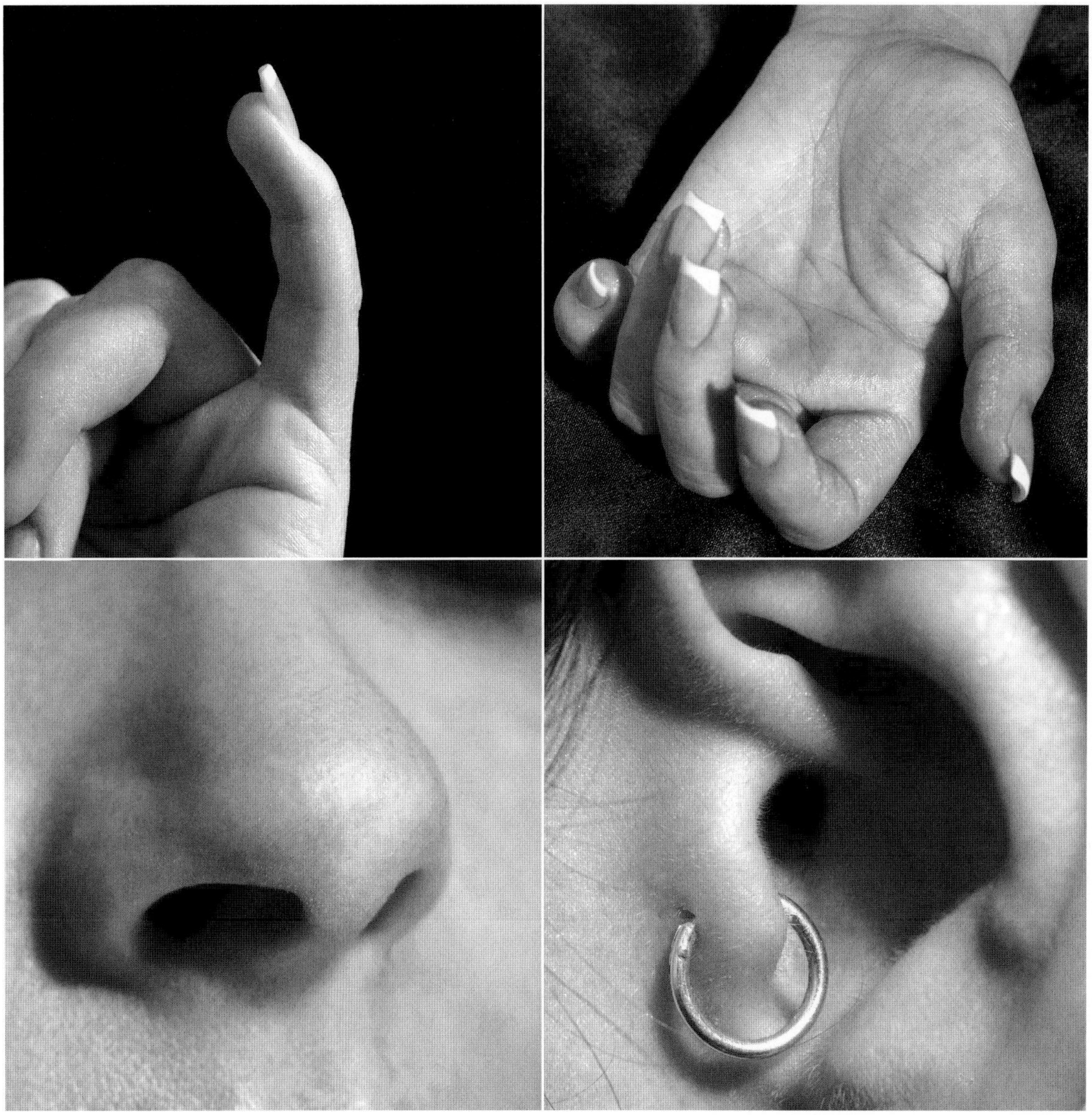

a b

c d

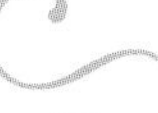

The Tertiary Erogenous Zones

The tertiary zones are:

- a The outside surface of the little finger
- b The center of the palm
- c The nostrils
- d The ear canal
- e The sole of the foot
- f The big toe
- g The back of the knee
- h The navel
- The anus

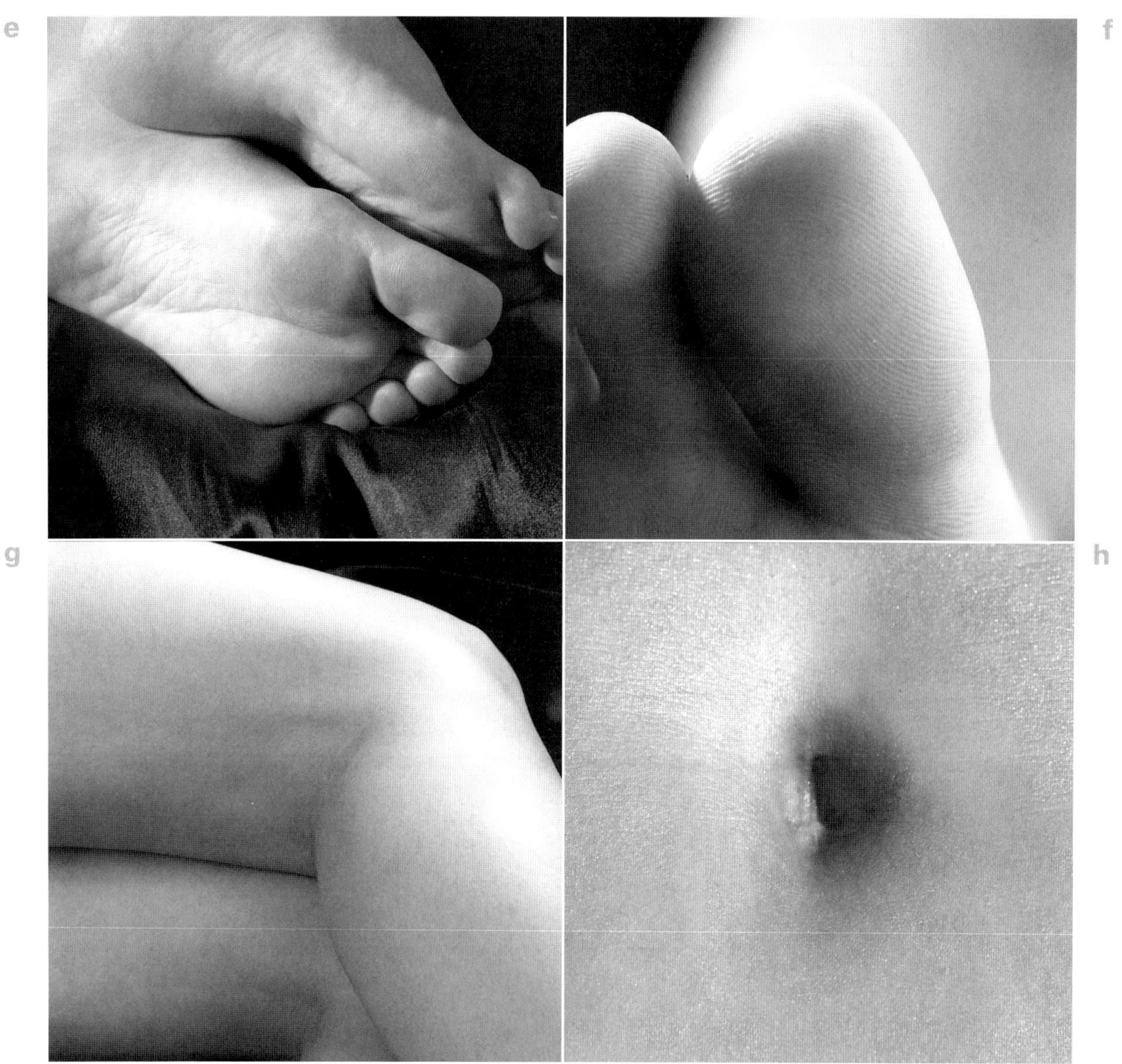

Become aware of where the erogenous zones are and the pleasure your partner experiences when you move from one to another. You will soon see your partner reach intense new levels of arousal.

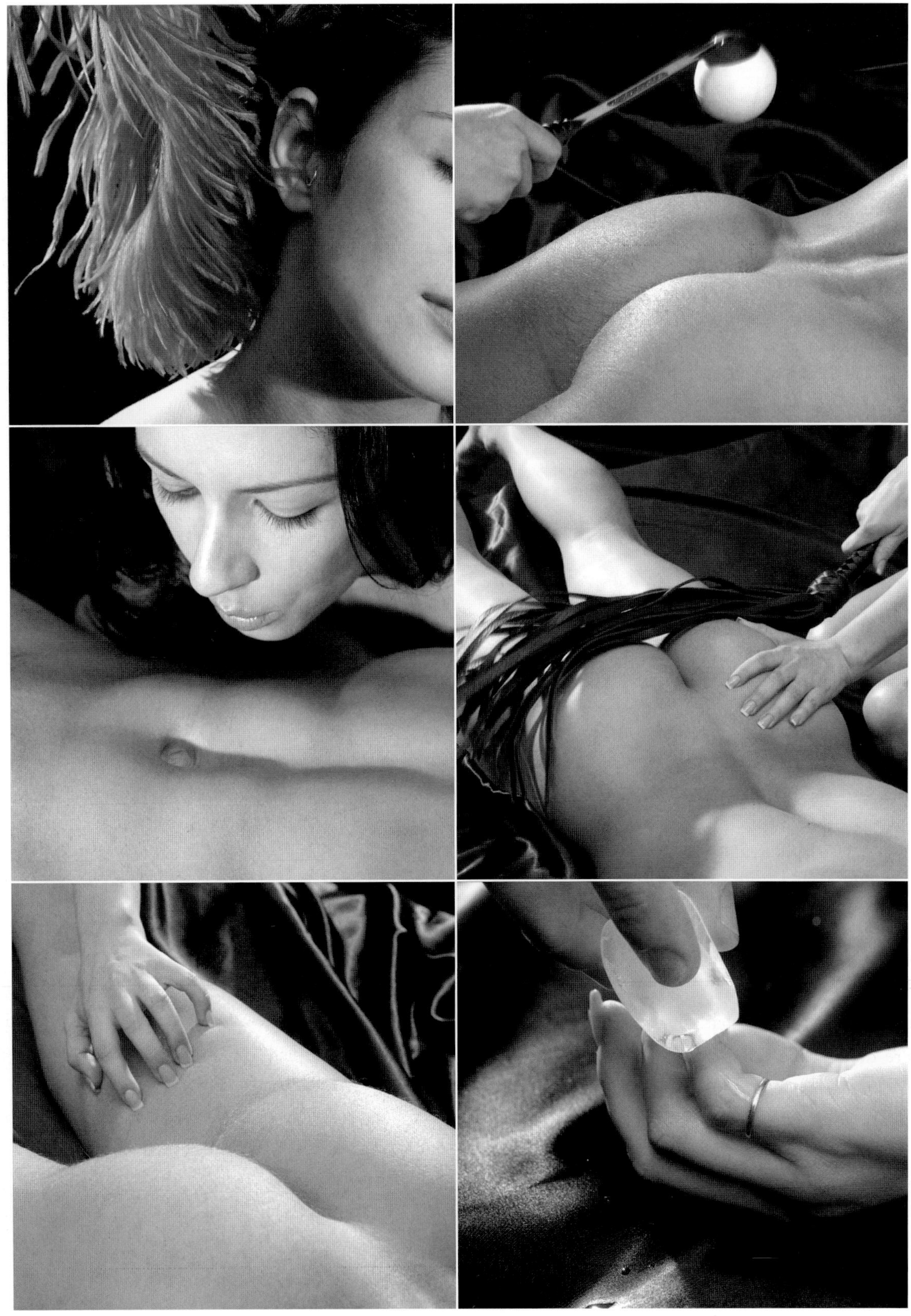

THE ART OF PLEASURING THE EROGENOUS ZONES

According to classical Indian sexual practice as translated by the noted author and scholar Dr. Jonn Mumford, the most effective way to stimulate these erogenous zones is in a four-beat pattern: first the secondary zones, then the primary zones (but not the genitals), then the tertiary zones, then back to the primary zones (including the genitals).

There are many ways you can do this. For example, you might stimulate *all* the secondary zones, then all the primaries (but not the genitals), then *all* the tertiaries, then go back to the primaries (minus the genitals). You might do this half a dozen times before you ever touch the genitals. Or you might kiss up the inside of a thigh (one secondary zone), then suck a nipple (one primary zone), then stroke the back of a knee (tertiary) while nibbling an earlobe (secondary), followed by a deep soul kiss on the mouth (primary).

To increase the arousal, start with the extremities and move in toward the genitals. For example, you can begin by biting the nape of the neck, then kissing a nipple. Move down the body with a two-handed, whole-hand-touching, gliding stroke until you reach the foot. Suck on the big toe, then lick your way up the leg to the back of the knee, where you can write "I love you" with your tongue. Follow with a teasing kiss on the mouth.

Do not get so caught up in the secondary/primary/tertiary/primary dance that you lose the point of what you're doing. The point is to drive your partner wild with pleasure, not to follow this pattern to the letter. Simply become aware of where the zones are and the pleasure your partner experiences when you move from one to anothe. You will soon see your partner reach intense new levels of arousal. In fact, you may actually see waves of pleasure rippling through the body in the form of little muscle twitches, vibrations, and shakes.

Although the most common way to stimulate the erogenous zones—and the entire body—is with your hands and mouth, there are an infinite number of other ways to provide pleasure. Combining harder and softer touches—all applied at your partner's resilient edge of resistance—keeps your partner alive, alert, and turned on. Pleasure-producing devices can be found throughout your house, as well as in sex shops and on the Internet. Here are just a few: a feather, fur, a silk scarf, a flogger, long fingernails, your breath, a ball massager, the Tingler (a flexible copper head massager), vibrators (of all types and sizes), an ice cube, long hair (stroked over the body), wooden spoons, Tiger Balm, a paddle, pickle tongs, clothespins, an electric toothbrush, a loofah sponge, a bath brush.

Precision Sense Focusing Device There is one more delicious pleasure creation I want to introduce you to before we begin our sensuous massage: Just for the fun of it, I call it the Precision Sense Focusing Device. The PSFD is a square yard of satin fabric with a 4-inch by 4-inch-square cut out in the center of it. You can easily make one at home. If you are handy with a needle, you can hem the raw edges, as well as the edges around the center square. If sewing isn't your thing, don't worry; just trim away any fraying edges. Place your PSFD anywhere on your partner's body and concentrate every bit of your attention on pleasuring those sixteen square inches of flesh. You can concentrate on one of the established erogenous zones, or you can create a new one!

OPPOSITE Combining harder and softer touches keeps your partner alive, alert, and turned on.

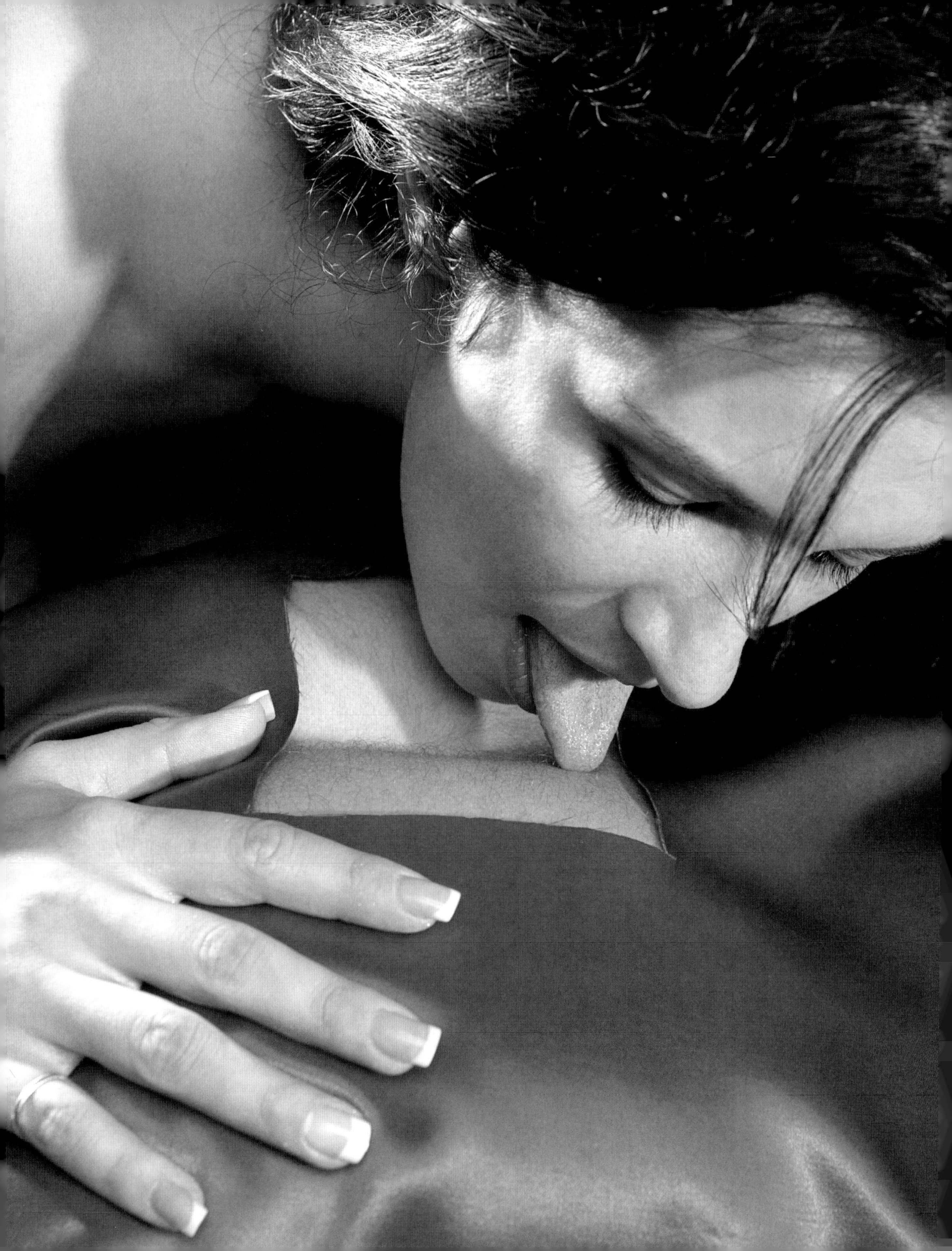

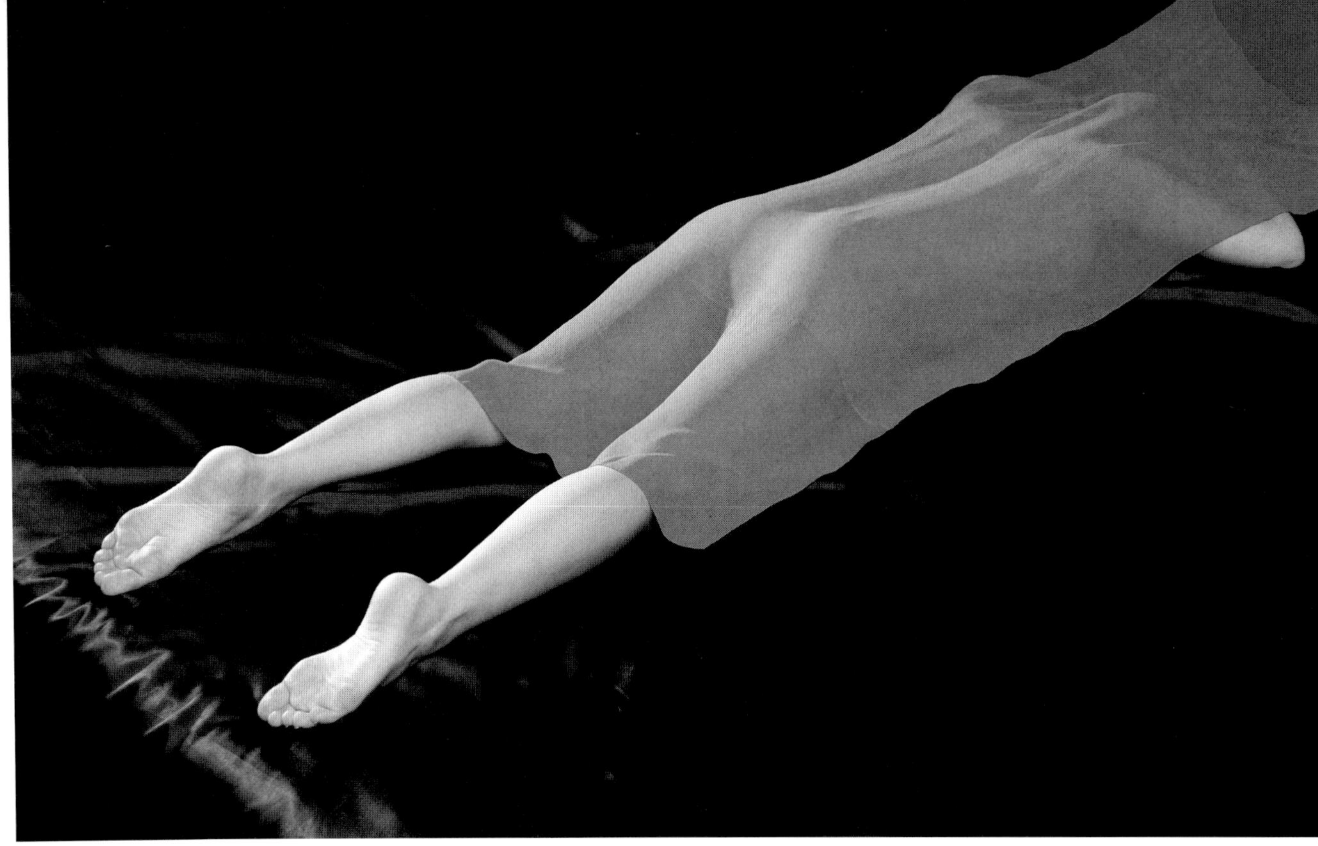

Create Your Own Sensual Massage

Now it's time for you to create your own sensuous massage. Remember, this massage is not about how skilled you are at massage therapy. It's about how deeply and consciously you can go into the process of giving your partner pleasure. If you are the person receiving the massage, try to release any expectations you may have about what will happen, what you will or won't feel, or how you are supposed to react. The art of receiving is simply breathing and staying aware of what you are feeling at each moment.

OPPOSITE The Precision Sense Focusing Devise, or PSFD

ABOVE Pull a silk scarf s-l-o-w-l-y over the body from feet to head.

Begin by deciding where you will be doing the massage. If you possibly can, buy yourself a massage table with adjustable legs. Although you can give a massage on the floor or on a bed, neither is the most comfortable height for the person giving the massage. It is hard to stay present and to give exquisite pleasure when your back is aching. If cost is a factor, you can always find used massage tables in the classifieds or on the Internet. Or ask at your local health-food store. A massage table is one of the best investments in pleasure you will ever make. If you don't have one right now, look around your house for a substitute. I have often used a dining-room table padded with a comforter and a sheet.

Gather any supplies you will need, such as sensual toys, your Precision Sense Focusing Device and a box of cornstarch (also known as cornflour). Cornstarch?! Absolutely. Try cornstarch instead of massage oil. It is

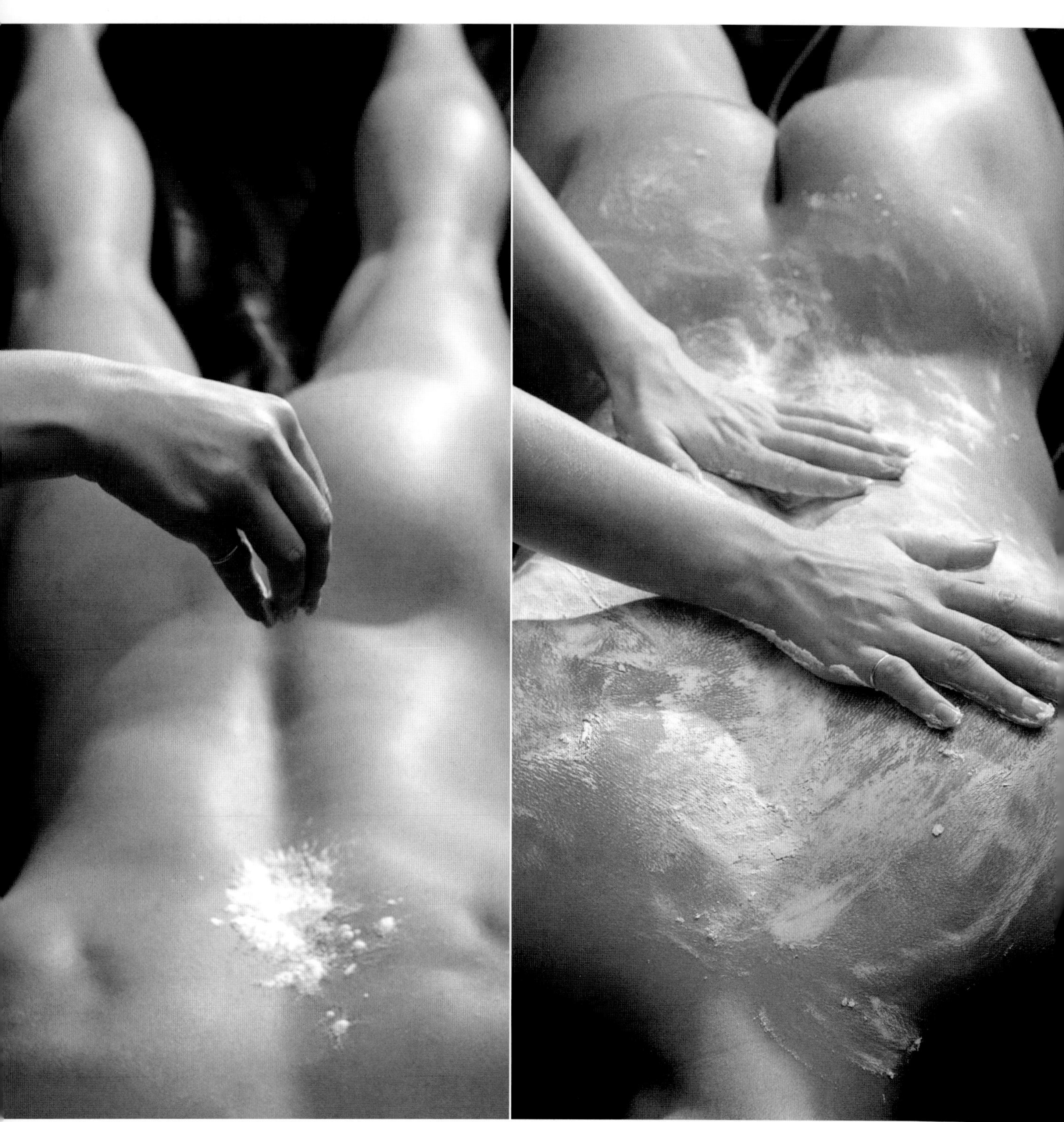

simply exquisite—it feels like powdered silk on the skin. It's also hypoallergenic and easy to clean up—just shake it out or vacuum it up.

Ask the receiver to lie facedown on the table. Begin with stillness. Place your hands—hearts of palms first—on your lover's body and breathe with him. Continue until you feel her breath drop into an easy rhythm. Then invite him to relax with a light full-body touch. Caress him from head to toe with an ostrich feather.

Or, holding a silk scarf in both of your hands, pull it s-l-o-w-l-y over his body from his feet to his head. Your intention is to help your partner relax and come to a deeper awareness of her body.

Now it's time to massage his entire body. Applying the cornstarch can be an elegant massage stroke all by itself.

With your fingers and thumb, pick up a generous dollop of cornstarch. Holding your hand twelve to eighteen inches above his body, let the cornstarch plop onto his back. It is a unique erotic sensation. He may moan, gasp, or giggle. You can do this several times. Then lovingly massage his back and front, from head to toe, with glides, kneading, vibrations, lifting and holding, and stillness. Remember to massage his hands, his feet, and his head—we carry so much tension in these places.

Now that he is relaxed and has come more deeply into his body, it is time to begin to bring in some more focused touch to begin to arouse him. (If you'd like to remove some of the cornstarch before continuing, you can use a towel or a soft brush to whisk it away.) This is where your knowledge of the erogenous zones and your collection of sensational toys (including your hands and mouth) come in. Keep in mind the resilient edge of resistance. You'll want to choose a sensation that awakens and energizes the body but does not assault it. For example, you could use a flogger at the gluteal fold (where the buttock meets the top of the thigh). Start slowly. You can always increase sensation as his arousal builds. Based upon how aroused he becomes with that stroke, you can judge how hard you'll kiss his mouth. If he has an intense reaction to that, you might want to surprise him by running an ice cube along the outside of his little finger —a subtle yet intense sensation. You could follow this by running your fingertips lightly over his penis. Then return to a more intense stroke, such as a bath brush at the base of his spine or a bite on his earlobe.

Very soon you will feel the dance of his arousal. All you have to do is keep dancing with him. Remember, the person receiving the massage is always in charge. You simply take your cues from your lover's reactions and his breathing. If you feel your attention lagging or you have an impulse to make something happen, move into stillness for a few moments. Just be. Allow the energy to run on its own (it will!). Match your breath to your lover's and then see where the dance leads you next.

Arousal has no limits except those that we create. Your partner may shake, moan, scream, giggle, laugh, cry, beg, or bliss out. Revel in it all. Support him with your touch and with sounds of encouragement. At the end of the sensuous massage, he may want to move on to intercourse or he may want you to bring him to orgasm. Or he may feel completely satisfied and move into deep meditation. If you stay focused on the excitement of the arousal rather than a climax, your sexual experience can become pure sensation and love, free from expectation or goal.

OPPOSITE Cornstarch feels like powdered silk on the skin.

Connect

CONNECT

10

I AM OCCASIONALLY ASKED BY SOMEONE who has heard a little bit about Tantra but has not practiced it, "What about fucking? Do you ever get to fuck?" Not only do you get to fuck but by making love as though fucking did not exist, everything begins to feel like fucking. You have been building enormous amounts of sexual energy with breath, eye gazing, movement, sound, taste, touch, and mindful awareness. By the time you get to intercourse, it already feels as if champagne bubbles are dancing under your skin.

When we do come together in genital union, we want to maintain our mindful awareness of the present moment. It is tempting to become goal-oriented as the energy builds. We certainly are not trying to avoid orgasm, but orgasm is not the goal. When we continue to focus on building arousal, we open the door to more intense, more ecstatic, more mind-blowing orgasms. Sex is energy and energy travels in circuits. When we come together in genital union, our bodies form the most intimate and powerful of energy circuits. Sensation is increased and energy is exponentially multiplied.

Origins of Sexual Positions

When you think of sexual positions inspired by Eastern traditions of sex, the Kama Sutra probably comes to mind. The Kama Sutra is the earliest surviving sexual how-to guide. Although widely spoken of today, the Kama Sutra was never meant to be a lover's guide for the general public. It was compiled for wealthy male city dwellers sometime between the second and fourth centuries CE. Although the Kama Sutra is best known for its in-depth discussion of sexual positions, only about 20 percent of the book is devoted to this. The rest contains advice about the acquisition of and

When we come together in a genital union, our bodies form the most intimate and powerful of energy circuits. Sensation is increased and energy is exponentially multiplied.

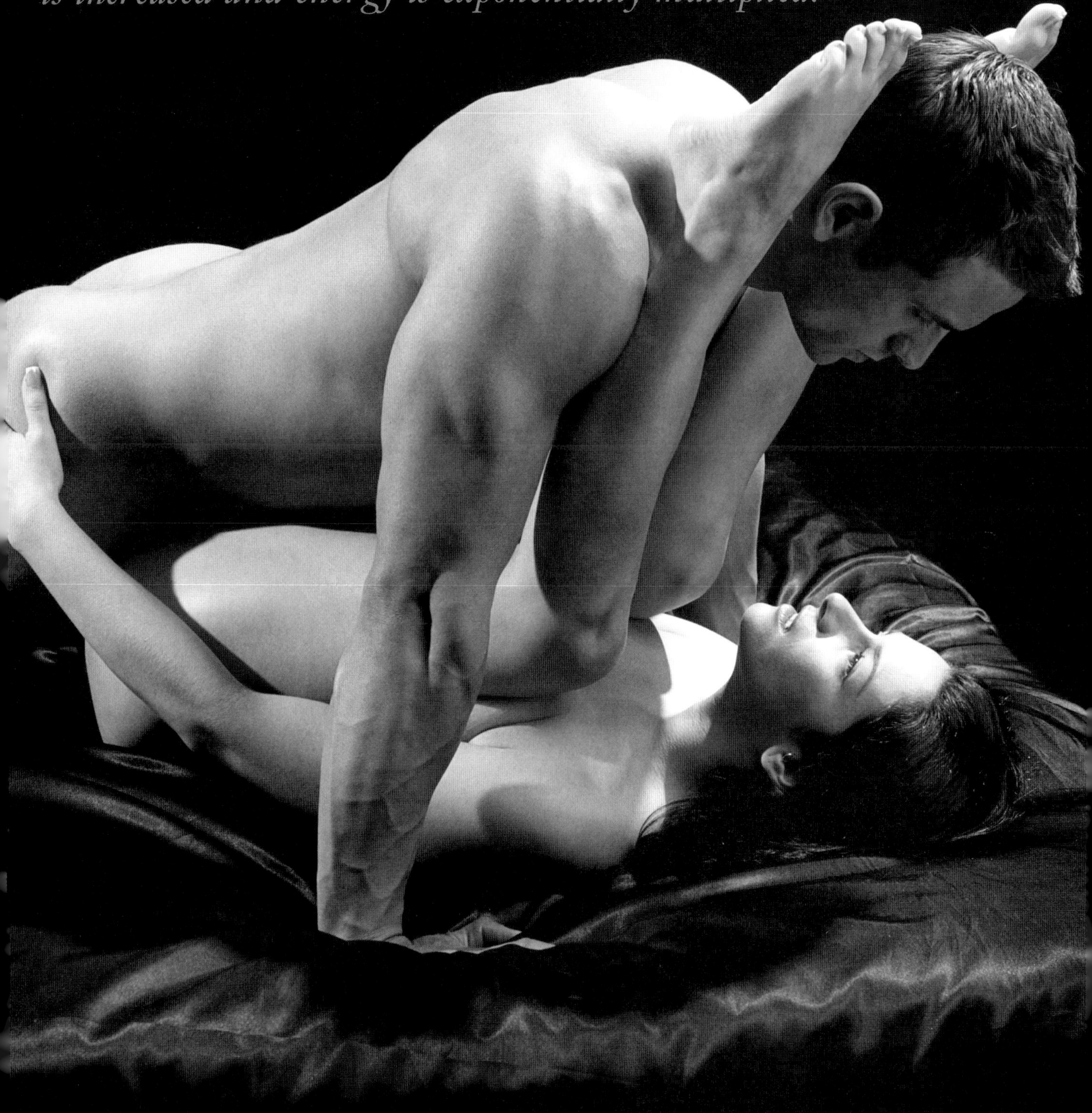

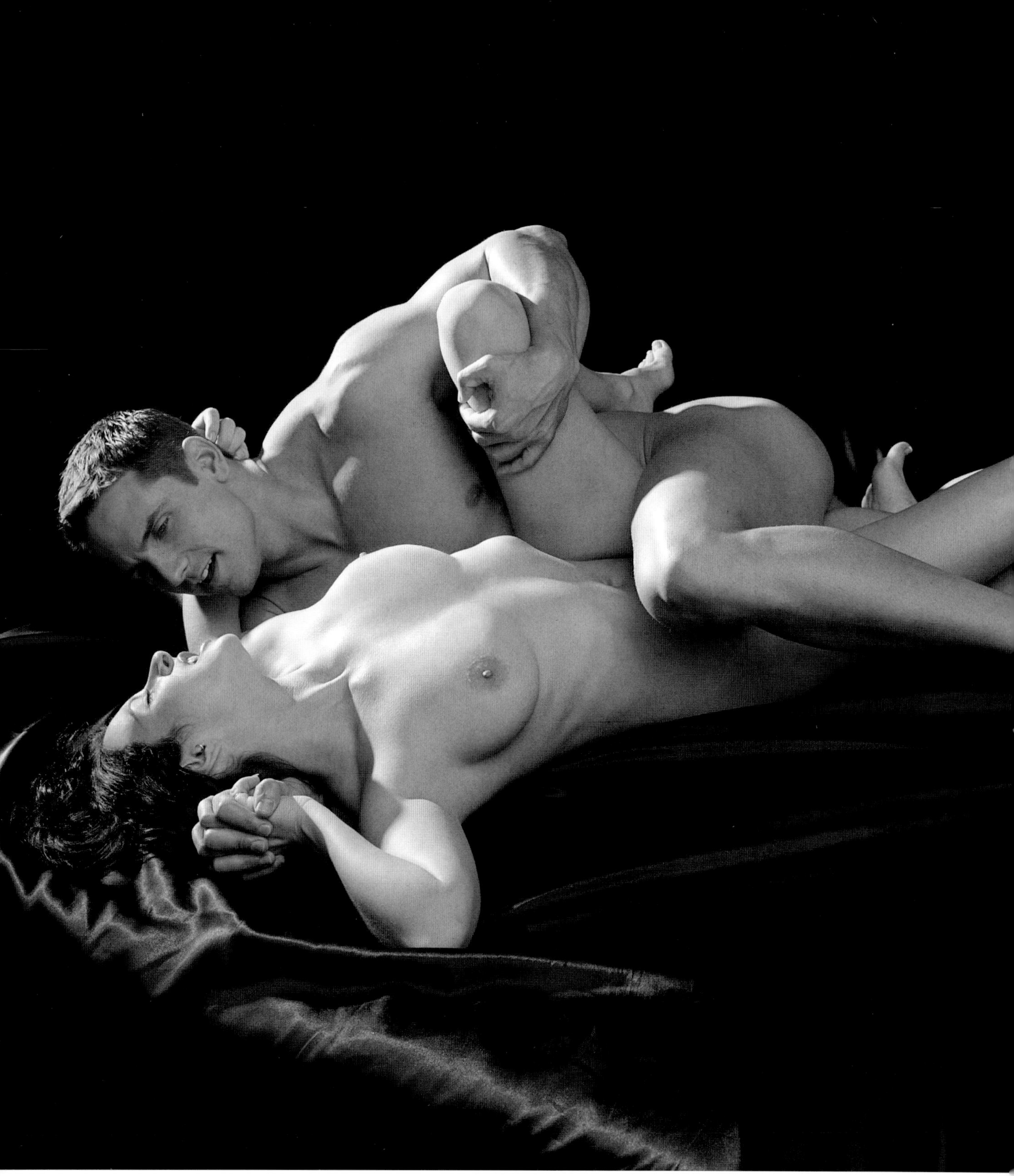

Key points of connection are the partners' eyes, hands, tongues, breasts, soles of feet, and genitals.

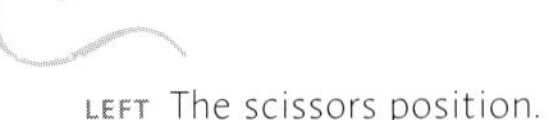

LEFT The scissors position.

proper conduct for a wife, the seduction of other people's wives, relations with courtesans, as well as advice on love in general and its place in the lives of men and women. The Kama Sutra is not a Tantric text, though over the centuries, some of the lovemaking positions have been reinterpreted in a Tantric way. It is easy to be intimidated by the number and complexities of sexual poses in the Kama Sutra. Many of these positions derive from hatha yoga, and, as in yoga, positions vary from the simple to the pretzelizing. All of these positions can be reduced to a manageable number of basic postures. The five basic lovemaking positions are:

1. Woman on top, man on his back;
2. Man on top, woman on her back;
3. Woman and man on their sides, facing each other;
4. Woman with her back to the man;
5. Seated positions, usually face-to-face.

Other positions are simply variations on a theme. The most important part of any posture is not how elaborately athletic it is but how well it facilitates the flow of sexual energy. Key points of connection are the partners' eyes, hands, tongues, breasts, soles of feet, and genitals. For example, look at the photo to the left.

SCISSORS POSITION

The scissors position is a variation of the side-by-side position. The lovers are connecting not only with their genitals but also with their eyes and hands, and their voices. There is nothing especially magical about this or any other position.

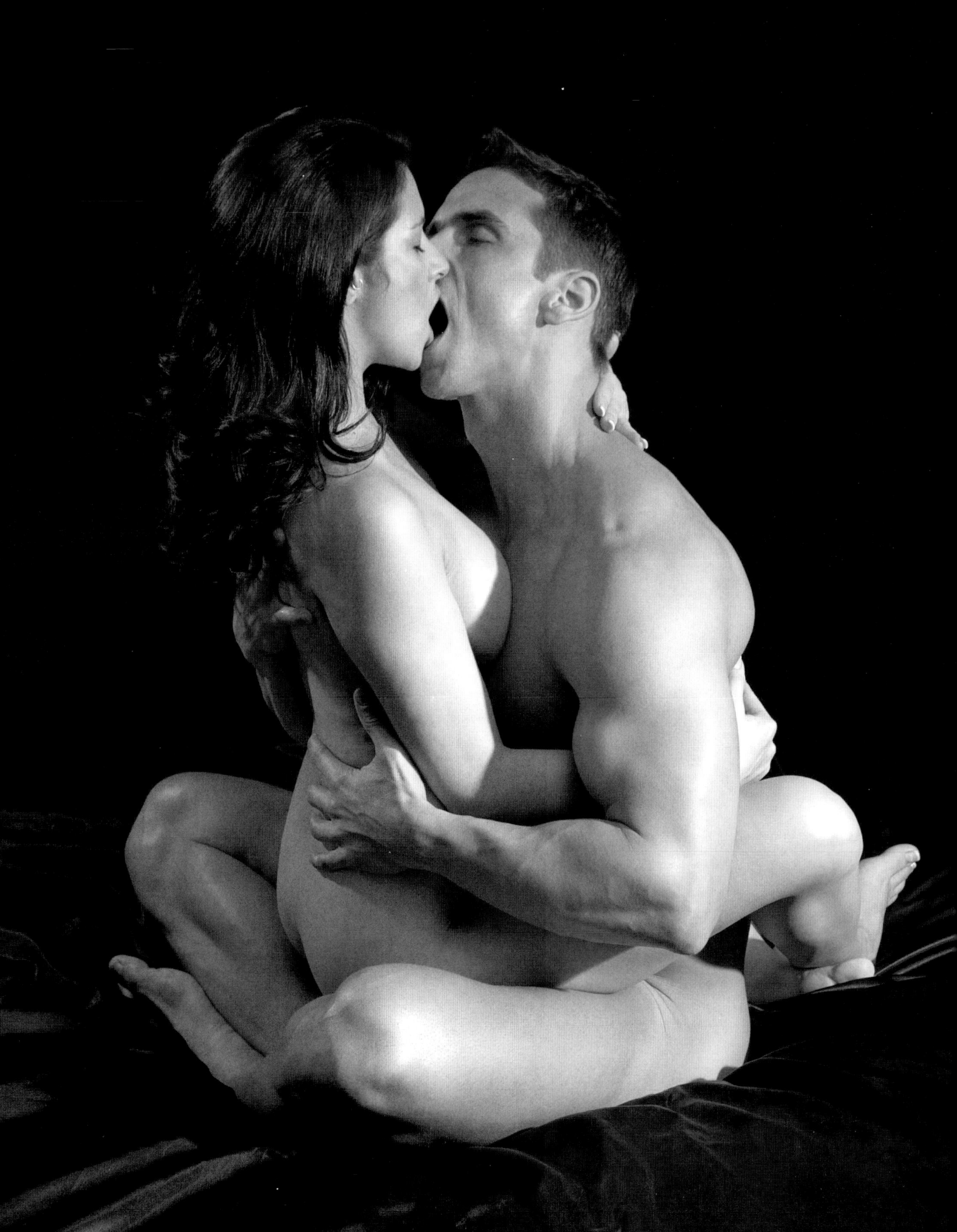

The magic comes from the mindfulness of the connection. Everything you do mindfully becomes a magical act. When you relax, when you go slowly and breathe, make sounds, maintain eye contact, and stay focused on what your body is feeling, the position in which you make love is unimportant. In Tantra, any position is potentially ecstatic when the lovers apply the practice of "three strokes for thirty," meaning it is better to make three conscious moves than thirty that are simply automatic and are not accom-panied by your total awareness.

YAB-YUM

The classic Tantric position, Yab-Yum, has many of the features we're looking for in terms of connection and the ability to stay mindful. Yab-Yum can be done with or without penetration. One partner (usually the man) sits in an easy cross-legged posture, with a cushion under his tailbone. The other partner (usually the woman) sits in his lap, with her legs wrapped around his waist and the soles of her feet touching. Both partners place their right hand at the back of their partner's neck and their left hand on their partner's tailbone.

In this position you and your lover are face-to-face and heart-to-heart. Yab-Yum is an awake, alive sitting position that allows sexual energy to move freely up the spine. You can breathe together, eye gaze or kiss, and the partner on top—usually the woman—has lots of opportunity to move. Yab-Yum often starts quietly and can build to intense levels of passionate activity.

OPPOSITE Yab-Yum with kiss.

TECHNIQUES FOR PROLONGING AROUSAL

There are several styles of lovemaking that illustrate the premise of three strokes for thirty. Many of these techniques require the man to delay (not deny) ejaculation. When the man delays ejaculation, lovers can stay in a virtually endless stage of arousal, floating in a mystical space of pure sensation and connection. In this realm, sexual positions and techniques become important not for their ability to produce orgasm but for their ability to produce prolonged, ever-increasing levels of physical delight and consciousness-altering bliss.

Karezza In karezza, the man moves only enough to keep his erection. A very pleasurable position in which to practice karezza is with the man on his back and the woman on top. In this position, she receives more stimulation—the natural curve of penis stimulates her G-spot—and he receives less intense stimulation, delaying ejaculation. She can keep him erect and both of them aroused with squeezes of her PC muscle. There may be moments of greater activity, followed by long restful periods. Both awareness and sensitivity are dramatically heightened. Karezza can lead to a state of "flowing" where preorgasm is indistinguishable from orgasm. After an hour or more of karezza, you cannot tell where you stop and your partner begins. You are both captured in a web of psychedelic timelessness. The secret to karezza is relaxation and lack of expectation. There can be no goal, only the reward of the bliss happening in each moment.

Pompoir is a powerful addition to any woman's sexual repertoire. In Pompoir, the woman flexes her vaginal muscles, gripping, massaging, and milking the penis. Developing the art of Pompoir is simple: regular Kegel exercises done every day for a few months. Once your

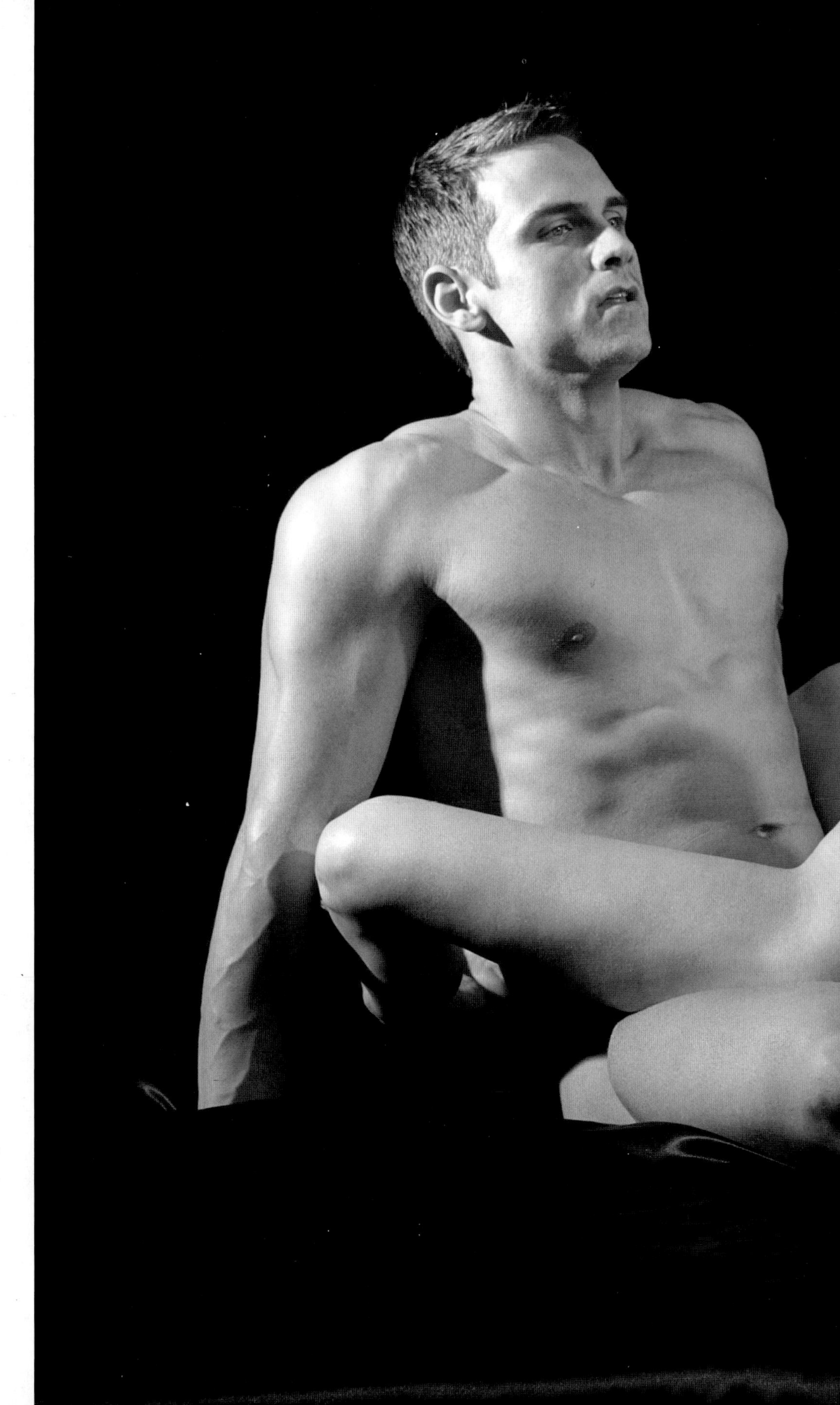

RIGHT Yab-Yum can build to intense levels of passionate activity.

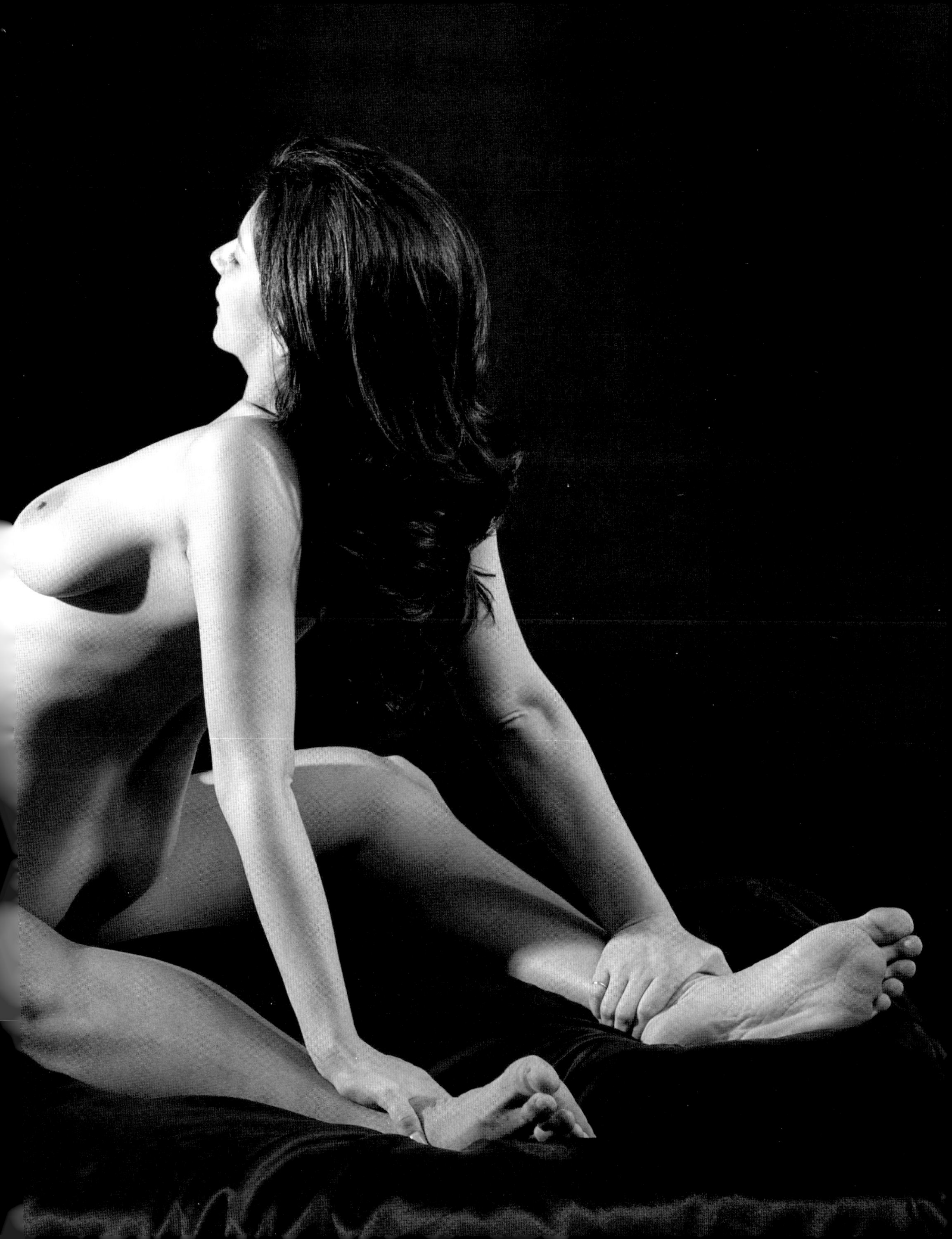

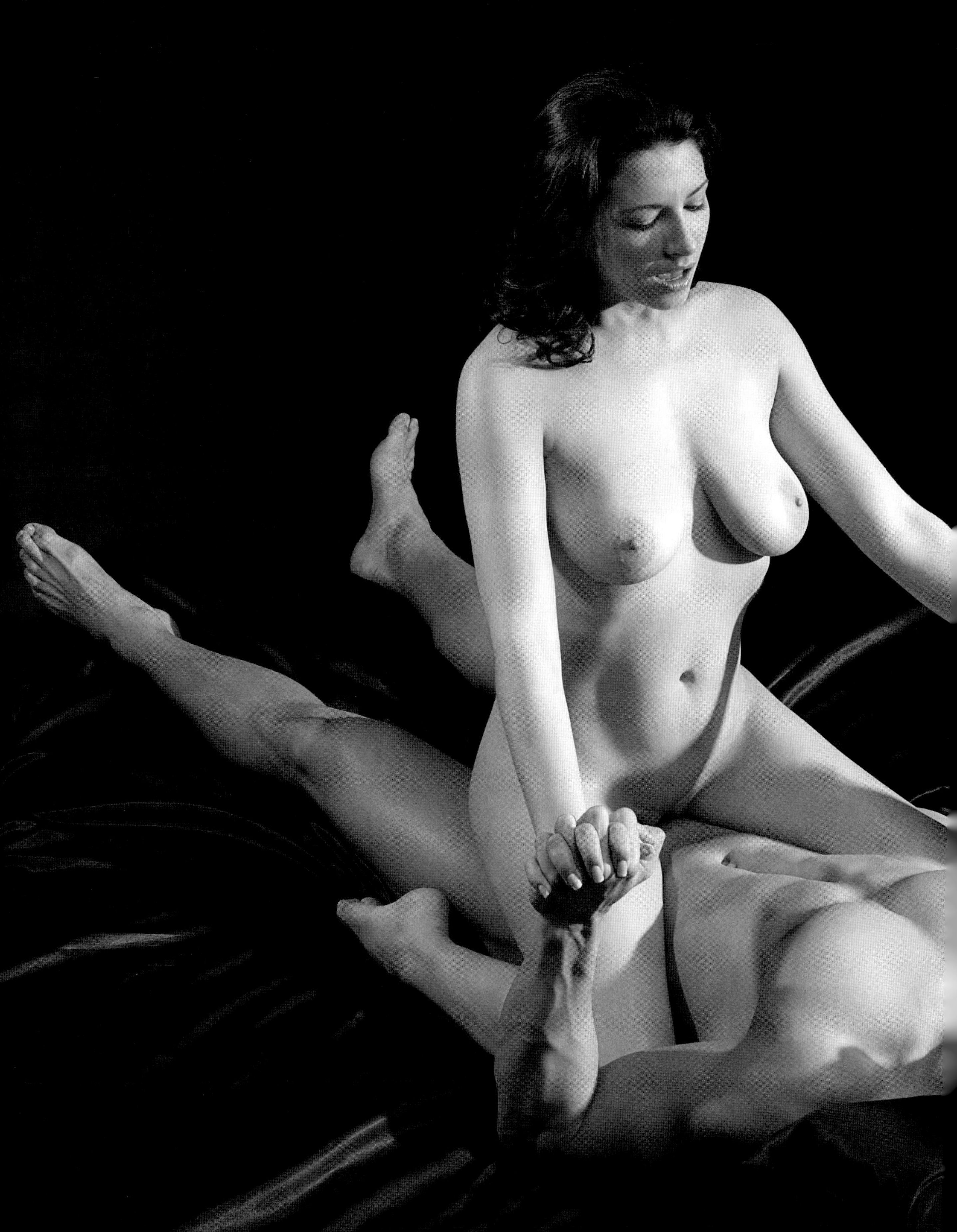

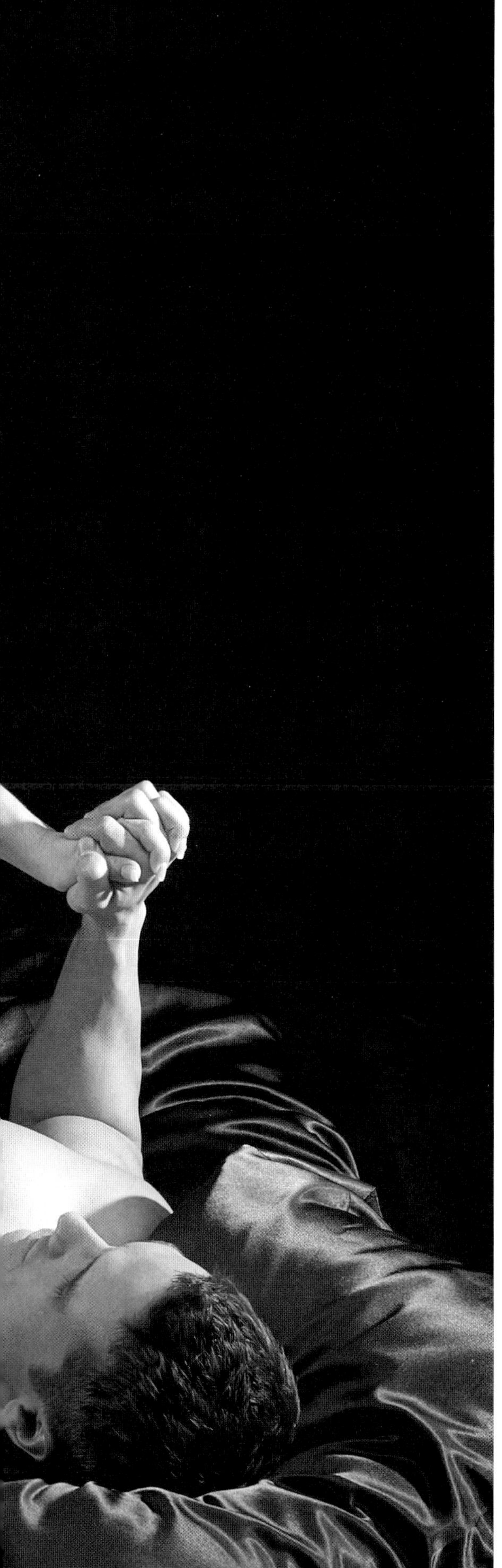

LEFT A very pleasurable position in which to practice karezza is with the man on his back and the woman on top.

PC muscle is in top shape, you can practice isolating different strands of the muscle, so that you grip deep inside the vagina as well as near the opening. This way you'll be able to massage different sections of the penis, producing the ancient milking skill known to the most talented sexual temptresses of ancient times.

Imsak is an ancient Arabian art in which a man thrusts slowly and withdraws his penis anytime he comes too close to ejaculation. With each successive penetration, arousal builds, until by the tenth union the ecstasy is mind-boggling. Most couples never reach anywhere near the tenth union, having found indescribable bliss long before that. The buildup of sexual energy is so intense that by the fifth union or so, a kiss seems to move the earth. In order to keep the energy building during the repeated cycles of penetration and withdrawal, equal attention must be paid to both the resting periods and the thrusting periods. During the rest periods, the man allows himself a few minutes of nonstimulation so that his erection and his need to ejaculate can subside. The woman may touch and caress him anywhere on his body except his genitals. This does not mean that the connection between the lovers becomes any less mindful, simply less genitally focused. Imsak allegedly was developed so that a man could satisfy a large percentage of his harem in one night. It was practiced with similar romantic success in the twentieth century by Prince Aly Kahn, whose father sent him to Cairo at the age of eighteen to learn the art of Imsak from the madams of the great Egyptian bordellos. The prince's legendary and countless romantic liaisons included a who's who of Hollywood royalty of his time, including Rita Hayworth, Zsa Zsa Gabor, Judy Garland, and Kim Novak.

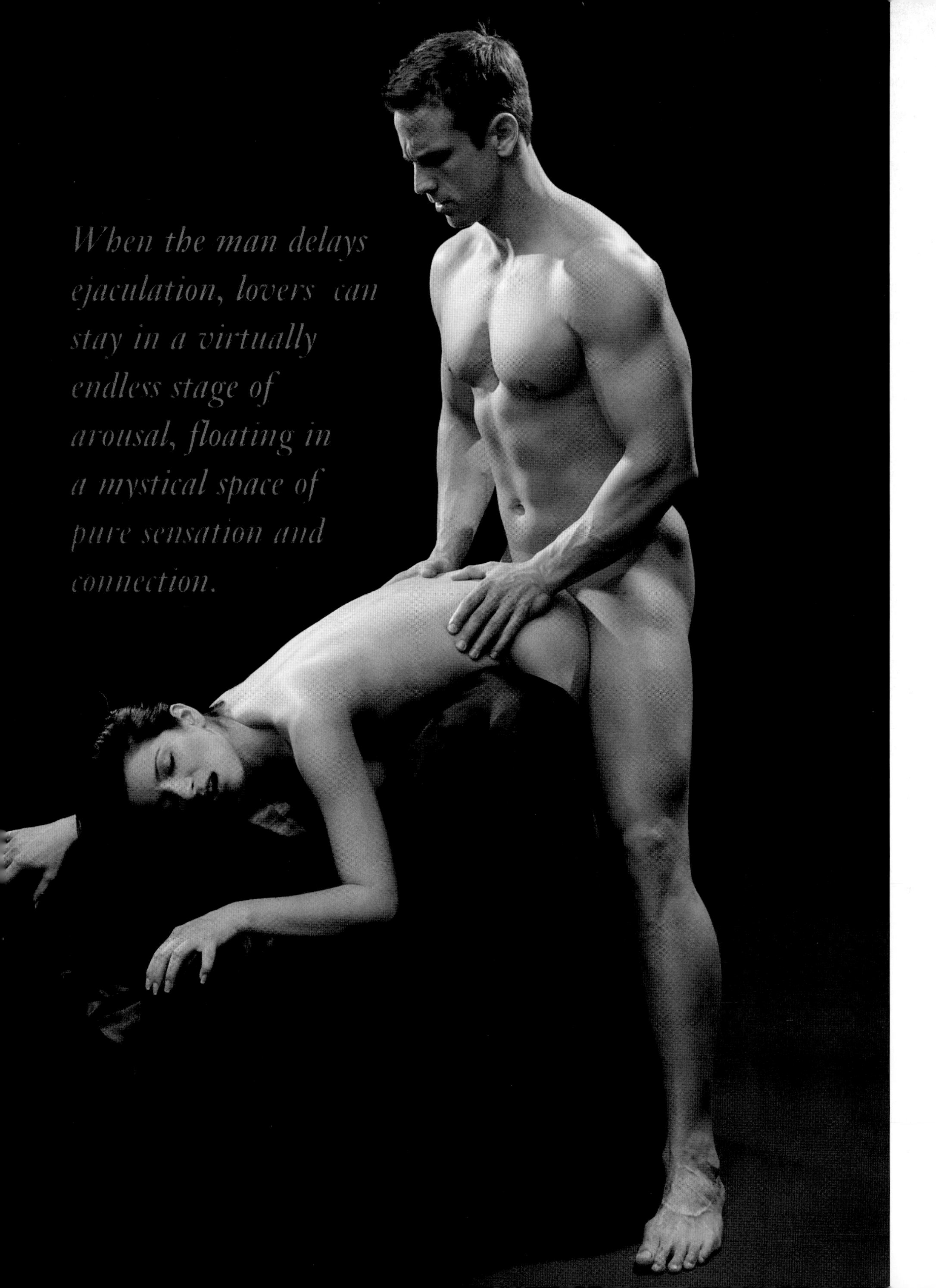

When the man delays ejaculation, lovers can stay in a virtually endless stage of arousal, floating in a mystical space of pure sensation and connection.

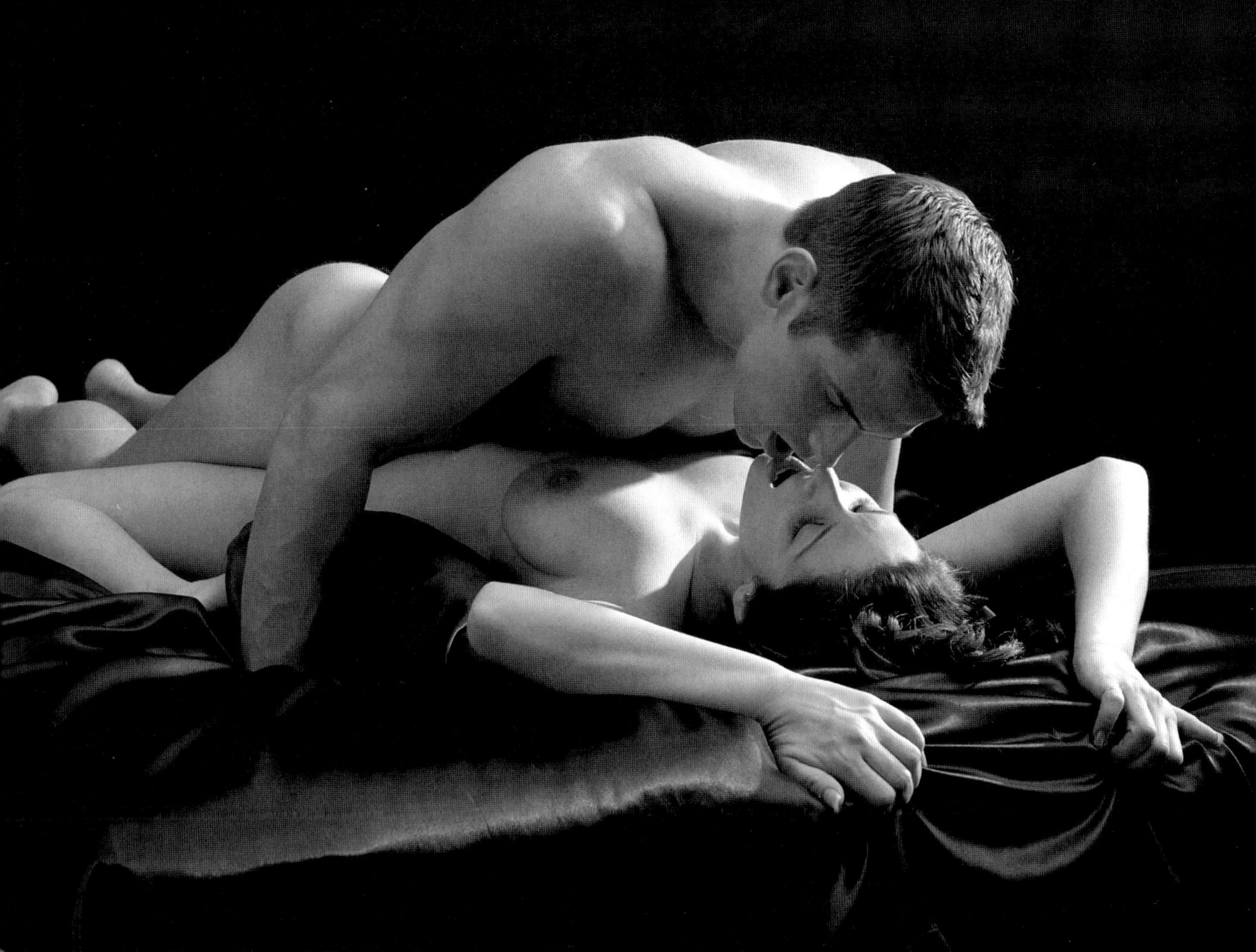

Thrusting is an art in itself. The three-strokes-for-thirty rule does not mean that thrusting should not be intense or deep or fast, though it should be none of these things exclusively. Variety is the key to intense arousal. Try this sequence, for example: First tease her clitoris with the tip of your penis before you enter her. When you finally do enter, stay just inside her, penetrating no farther than with the head of your penis. When you do move, thrust with a rhythm. Try three or six or nine shallow strokes, followed by one deep thrust. Your partner will inevitably pick up this rhythm and greet your thrusts with some of her own. Be creative. Compose your own unique patterns and rhythms. Remember, it is possible to stay connected and mindful even in high-energy poses if you start off consciously and focus not on orgasm but on building sexual energy.

Oral Sex is another wonderful way to build sexual energy while giving your partner intense pleasure. Instead of trying to give your partner an orgasm, approach oral sex as a tasting and caressing exercise. Use your hands as well as your mouth. In Chinese tradition, fellatio is called playing the flute because of the delightful part fingers play in stroking and massaging the penis.

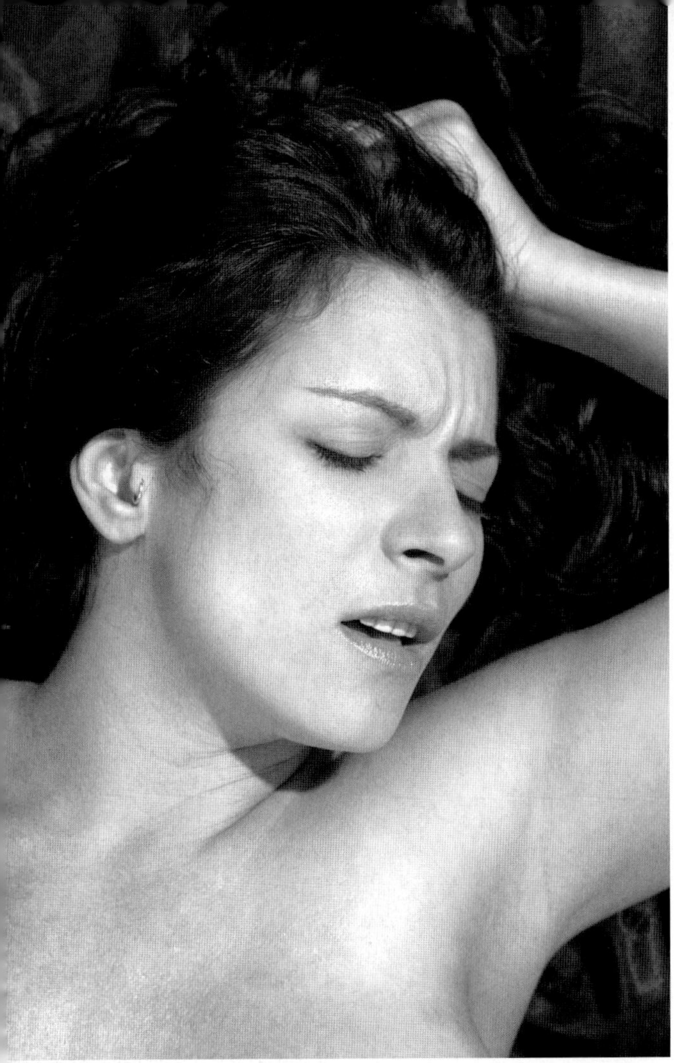

Your fingers can play an equally important part in cunnilingus. Pretend that your lover's vulva is a precious, pearl-laden oyster and open it with your fingers and tongue. Remember that sexual energy only starts in the genitals. As you pleasure your lover's genitals with your mouth, spread that energy all through his or her body with your hands.

Simultaneous oral sex, or 69, is a delicious circuit of pleasure. Visualize sexual energy traveling from your mouth to his cock, then up his body to his mouth, into your vagina, then up your body and into your mouth. Build the energy with your mouth, then move it around by visualizing this circuit and by stroking your partner's body with your hands. Concentrate on building the energy as if the two of you were one organism. Do not try to make anything happen—simultaneous orgasm is not the goal here. Simply feel the energy in the circuit and allow that energy to increase.

Think Implosion, Not Explosion

This luxurious, goalless style of connecting is like surfing a wave. You want to stay on the part of the wave where the energy is strongest. When you are on the face of the wave, energy is constantly building and carrying you forward. If you are too far in front of the wave, trying to make something happen before you have built up sufficient momentum, the energy is low. If you lose control and fly over the top of the wave, the ride is over. When men resist the temptation to ejaculate as soon as possible, they can ride the sexual wave indefinitely and are rewarded with intense new levels of pleasure. This also benefits the woman, who usually takes longer to build the same amount of sexual energy. The longer men take to build arousal, the more sensitive they become to the subtler nerve currents that control the ejaculation reflex. Ejaculation becomes a choice, not a reflex.

It is possible for men to experience orgasm without ejaculation. Orgasm without ejaculation feels like an implosion, rather than an explosion. Some men describe the experience as a huge expansion building up from deep inside them. When a man learns how to orgasm without ejaculating, he is capable of multiple orgasms. Men who have not yet experienced orgasm without ejaculation may suspect that ejaculationless orgasms are something less than a "real" orgasm. In fact, it's a very advantageous trade-off. As one practitioner of voluntary ejaculation put it, you have to be willing to give up the last ten seconds of the normal sexual climax cycle in order to experience the rest of it over and over again.

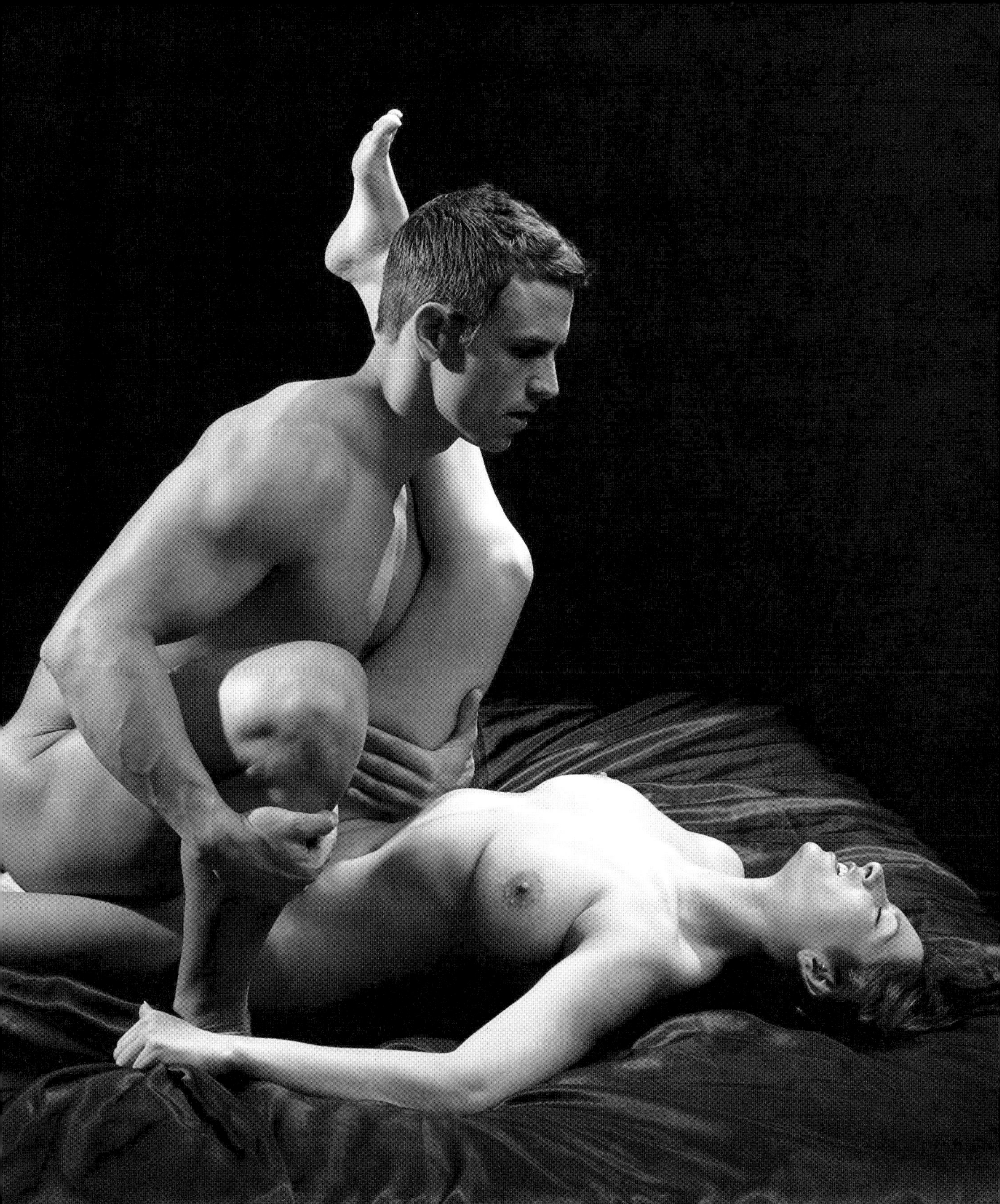

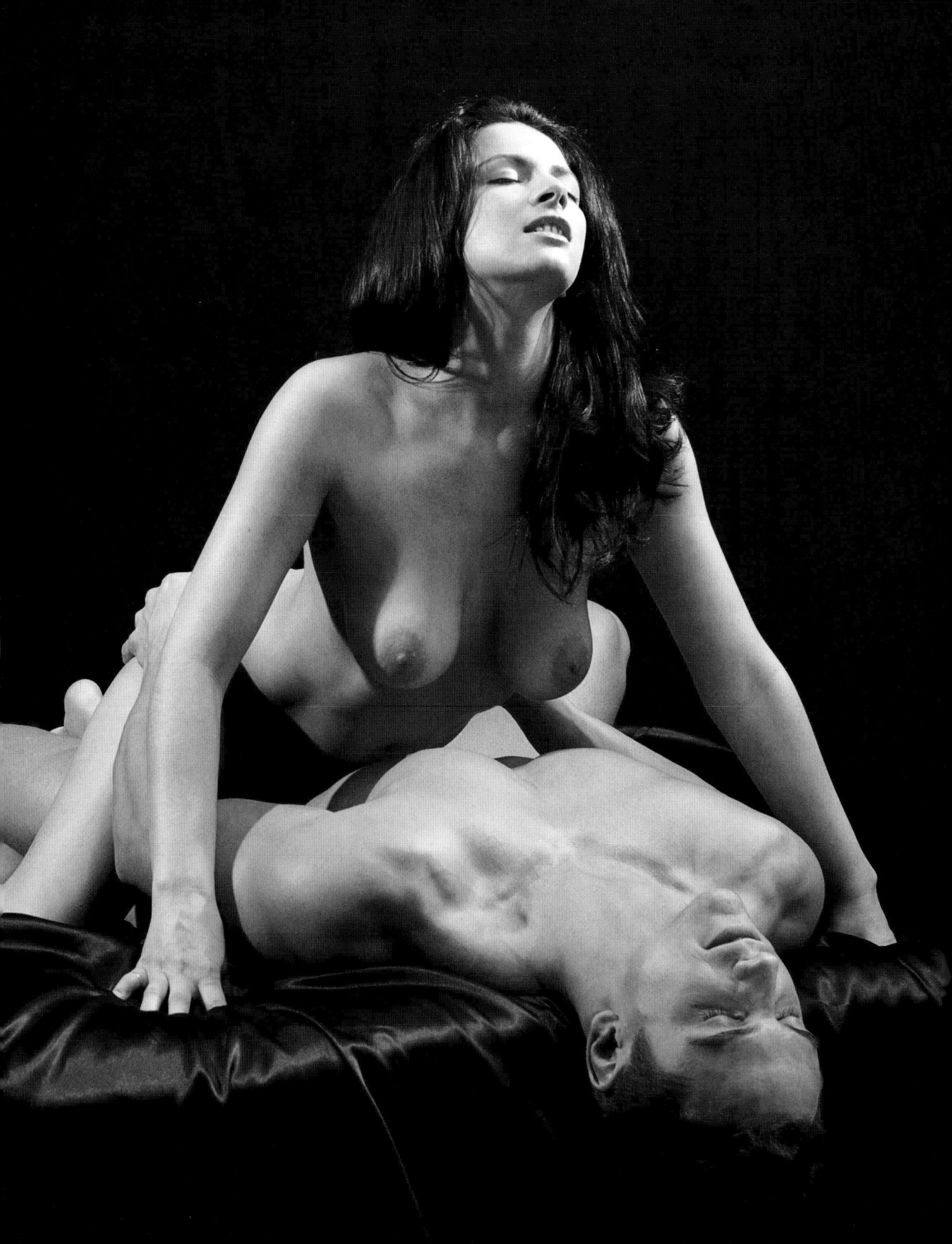

STAY RELAXED

Relaxation is the key to voluntary ejaculation. Most men have learned how to achieve orgasm under stressful situations. Adolescents learn to ejaculate as quickly as possible to avoid being caught in the act of masturbation, and often a man's first sexual experiences with a partner are similarly rushed. Now that you are an adult, you'll need to relearn orgasm in order to experience the extended possibilities of pleasure available to you and your lover. You do not have to do the multiplication table in your head to avoid ejaculation. When you use tricks like this to distract yourself, you become a spectator instead of a mindful participant in lovemaking. This trick fails most of the time, anyway. Instead, you need to gain control of your PC, anal, and urethral muscles that must contract for ejaculation to occur. You can easily feel your PC and anal muscles when you do a Kegel, and you can easily strengthen these muscles by doing daily Kegel exercises. It's more difficult to sense and develop control over spasmodic involuntary contractions of the smooth muscles of the prostatic urethra—the tube that begins at the bladder, passes through the prostate and exits at the tip of the penis. Advanced Kegel exercises will help you identify these smooth muscles. Once you have strengthened your PC and anal muscles, you can begin to Kegel on a deeper level. As you Kegel, breathe and imagine the inside of your penis. (You might want to look up the prostatic urethra on the Internet or in an anatomy book to get a picture of what you're trying to feel.) Follow that tube. Develop a feeling of it. Meditate on it as you squeeze and let go. For extra feeling, sit on a rolled-up towel; the nerves of the pelvic floor are sensitive to pressure. With practice, patience, and focus, you will be able to recognize and control these smooth muscles.

PRACTICE ON YOURSELF

Next, practice voluntary ejaculation while masturbating. Give yourself at least twenty minutes. Masturbate almost to the point of orgasm. As you approach orgasm, notice what is happening in your body. What muscles are you tensing? How are you breathing? What are you doing that is speeding up ejaculation? Now, just as you are on the verge of orgasm, go from profound contraction to profound relaxation. Go totally limp, completely soft inside. During this moment of relaxation, take your focus off your genitals. Direct it to the top of your head or your Third Eye. You'll feel your orgasmic energy remain in motion, even though the muscles of your genitals are not. Sexual energy will go wherever you put your attention. If you focus on stopping your penis from having an orgasm, your focus is still on your penis, so that's where the energy will flow and you will ejaculate. Remember that your most powerful pleasure center is your brain. Direct your orgasm there and you will experience pleasure while your genitals cool down. If you practice these exercises regularly, within a couple of months—or sooner—you will be having multiple orgasms. Remember, the trick is learning to stay relaxed in high states of arousal. This is easier to learn in passive, receptive mode. You can't relax the smooth muscles of the urethra while you're thrusting, so when you're with your lover, lie back and let her get on top. Let her be the surfer and you the surfboard. Relax, breathe, and slow down.

Please remember that sex is fun! Don't let yourself become overwhelmed, put off, or obsessed by any one position or technique. Sexual techniques exist only as pathways to pleasure. Enjoy the journey. Along the way you'll visit lots of ecstatic, awesome, fulfilling destinations. When you share the journey with your partner, you'll find that your relationship, your lovemaking, and your lives will all become magically transformed.

Imagine

IMAGINE

11

In the first chapter, you imagined what your sex life would be like if it could be as luxurious as a five-star hotel. In the chapters that followed, you read about—and (I hope) experimented with—a variety of erotic luxuries that have helped you intensify and expand your pleasure in the arousal phase of love-making. You may already have begun to relax into the fantastic natural high of intense arousal and expanded orgasm during which magical things appear to happen:

- You may feel as if you are flying.
- You may scc bright colors or fccl that your body is a single ecstatic organ.
- You may be able to "read" your lover's thoughts.
- You may even feel as though you have disappeared.

Once you start to experience these extraor-dinary occurrences, more and more of them will happen for you. You'll even start seeing magical things happen in other areas of your life. You may feel more alive, more aware, and unusually lucky, as though the universe is conspiring on your behalf. Magic does not happen haphazardly. Neither does luck or happiness or bliss. Good things happen to us because on some level we expect them to happen. Why is it, for example, that one person will look down at the ground and find a hundred-dollar bill, while two dozen other people will step over that same bill and not see it? The person who sees the hundred-dollar bill believes on some level that it is possible to receive one hundred dollars with little or no effort. His view of how the universe works includes the possibility of a hundred-dollar bills appearing at his feet. To him, this magical event is simply the logical affirmation of his beliefs.

Expanded Awareness and Visions

Similarly, it will become just as natural for you to experience—and accept as both logical and natural—an expansion and elevation of awareness that some people describe as holy or sacred. One of the most common manifestations of this expanded awareness is seeing visions, usually during states of high arousal or in the afterglow of an orgasm. Some visions may be mystical and otherworldly, while others may offer practical information. At first you may question the information you

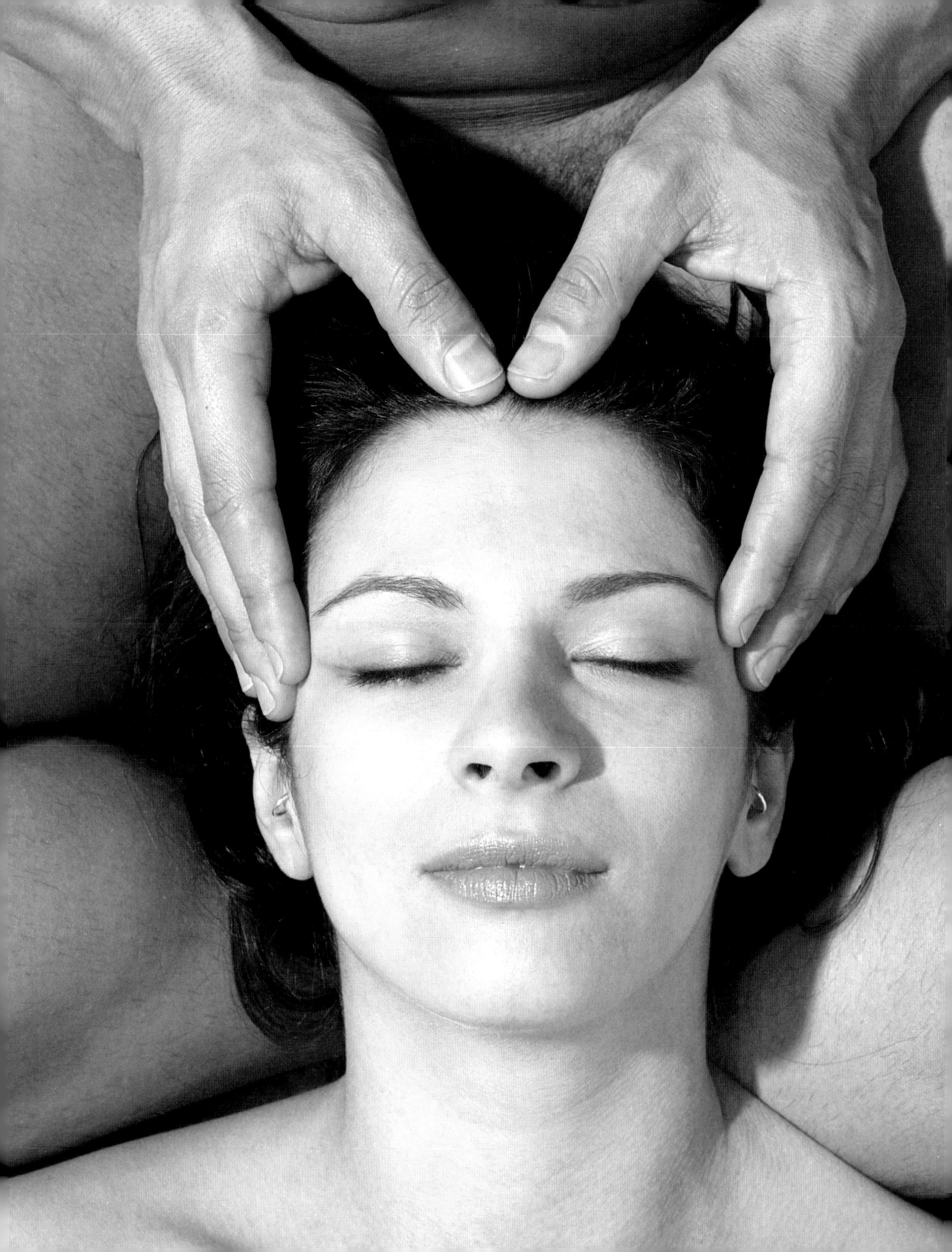

receive in these visions. You may wonder if the visions are "real" or just figments of your imagination. They could be both. Some visions are received as revelations; others are created with your imagination.

Visions that appear to be revelations are no different from other unseen and unspoken messages that you receive every day. We each have our own personal antenna that picks up signals from the unseen world. Your antenna picks up bits of information and translates them into what you could call gut instinct or hunches. You may have an unexplainable inclination to walk down one street rather than another, or you may stop in at a local café because you have a hunch a friend may be there. During a high state of sexual arousal, your antenna becomes more alert. The signals you receive are more than hunches; they are the callings of your soul or the whisperings of a higher power.

Sometimes visions, like dreams, come in symbolic form. For example, you may have the feeling that you are being offered some kind of gift by the universe, but you don't know what the gift might be. This is when your imagination is useful in interpreting the feeling. Ask yourself, "If I knew what this was, what would it be?" Then let your imagination answer. For example, if you knew who was offering the gift, who would it be? An image of a person or animal offering you a gift in a box might pop into your mind. Then you could ask again, "If I knew what this gift was, what would it be?" When you open the box, you may see an image that reveals to you that you are being given good health, prosperity, or the answer to a question that has been in your mind for some time.

Some visions are created entirely by your imagination. These are just as important, valid, and real as the visions that appear to come from "nowhere." You can use your imagination to create a vision of a better relationship, a bigger home, or world peace. The more you concentrate on these visions, the more likely they are to materialize. To make any desire materialize, you first must believe it is possible. The job, the house, and the car you have now were at one time desires that you first imagined, then created. Once you have the things you once desired, you create new preferences and begin to imagine new desires, which in turn create new experiences. In this way, you can imagine and then make real any relationship or sex life you like.

Sex Magic

One of the most enjoyable and powerful uses of your imagination and your sexuality is sex magic. Sex magic is the art of transforming real but invisible sexual energy into real and visible results. You have already practiced one type of sex magic in chapter 1, when you focused all your attention on the index finger of your right hand and felt your finger grow bigger, tingly, and warmer. You practiced it again in chapter 2 when you used your imagination and your breath to bring sexual energy from your genitals to your heart. Both of these are solid demonstrations of energy following thought.

Sex magic is what happens when you put your sexual energy where your intentions are. You can use sex magic to connect with a higher power, to direct healing energy to yourself or to someone else, or to influence the outcome of a given situation. Sex magic is not religion, though it can certainly feel like a physical prayer. What makes sex magic different from other types of magic or prayer is the sheer power of the erotic. When you are in a high state of sexual excitement, enormous quantities of energy are released in the body, producing a trancelike state of consciousness in which you may feel egoless and without boundaries—as if you are part of everything that exists. When you are in this hypnotic state of sexual excitement, you become especially receptive and impressionable. Visions you hold—and words you hear—at this time are powerfully imprinted on your consciousness. (This is why partners need to be especially aware of what they say to each other during lovemaking.) This combination of energy and receptivity offers a unique opportunity for transformation.

SIMPLE STEPS FOR PRACTICING SEX MAGIC

Sex magic is as simple as it is powerful. It can be effectively practiced in just four easy steps:

1. Have a vision of your goal. Be sure to visualize what you want—not what you don't want. If you want to send sex magic to bring peace to a war zone, for example, don't create a vision of dead soldiers and bleeding civilians. Rather, envision a stable, happy population brimming with goodwill and prosperity. You can be really corny and unsubtle about this—envision everyone hugging and counting large sums of money. If you simply can't manage to hold on to a completely positive vision, create a symbol to represent your vision, such as a peace sign or a heart.
2. Hold your vision in your mind for a few moments before you begin to raise sexual energy.
3. As you begin to raise sexual energy, let go of your vision. Forget about it. Concentrate instead on your body and your pleasure.
4. At orgasm, or at the peak of your arousal, flash on your vision for a few seconds. Imagine a huge movie screen in your mind and let your vision flicker on and off, on and off. This helps imprint the image more deeply in your unconscious.

That's all it takes to begin your practice of sex magic. You can do it alone or with a partner. You can create solo masturbation rituals that incorporate other kinds of magic. Some people make an altar, using power objects; or they call in the four elements (earth, air, fire, and water) or the four directions. None of that is necessary, but ritual practices such as these do serve to create a space and time that separates your sex-magic ritual from the rest of your life.

Try a solo sex-magic ritual for yourself. Perhaps you would like to lose weight or stop smoking or start an exercise program. Before you begin your self-loving, see yourself as a happy, healthy, slim, fit nonsmoker. Make your vision as rich and specific as you can. How would it look, feel, taste, smell, and sound to be this happy, healthy, slim, fit nonsmoker? Once you have your vision, let it go. Focus your attention and intention on building as much sexual energy as you can. Use a fantasy to make your self-loving even hotter. As you are about to orgasm, flash on your vision. Keep the image flashing as you orgasm and for a few seconds after. Some people meditate on their goal again in the afterglow.

The energy you raise with sex magic can be as easily directed outward as inward. It is just as easy and possible to send healing energy to someone at a distance as it is to send sexual energy throughout your body or enlist it for your own self-transformation.

USES FOR SEX MAGIC

The idea of influencing outcomes at a distance may seem improbable to you. However, scientific studies have shown that prayer, or directed thought, has been shown to have a discernible positive effect on everything from heart patients to seeds in the ground to microorganisms. Even if you do not believe that your sexual energy can have any effect on someone across town or across the country, keep in mind that thinking you can do or have something is the first step in making it happen. When you are able to hold the vision of a friend as healthy, happy, and prosperous, you will treat him as healthy, happy, and prosperous when you next see him a

b

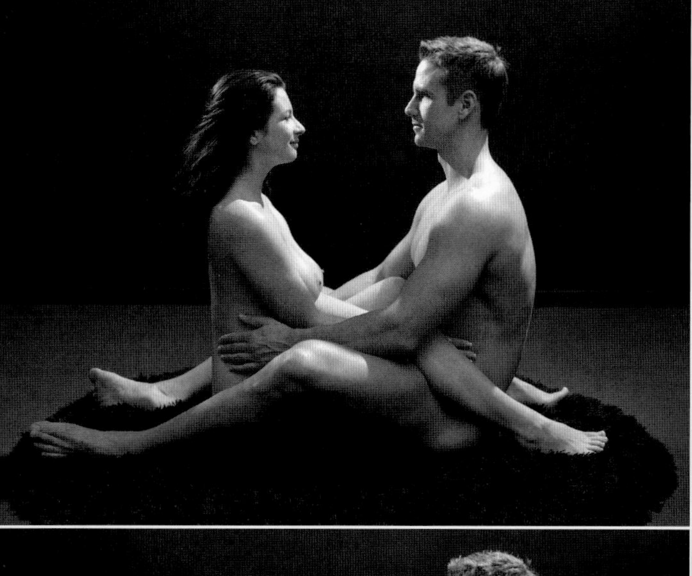

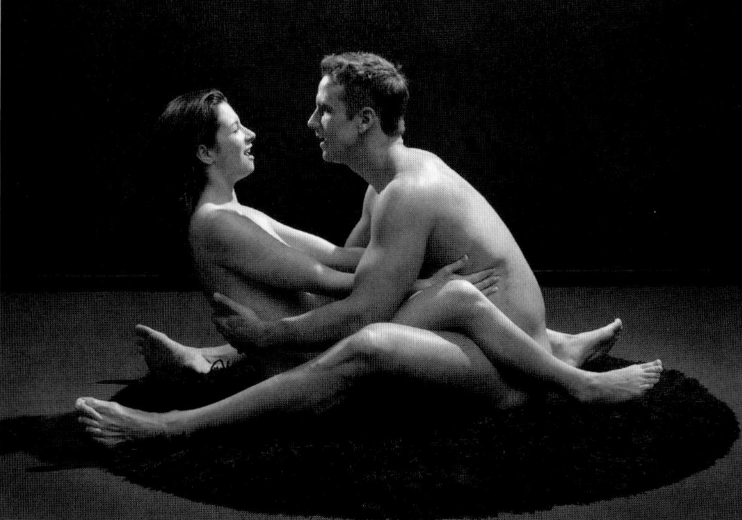

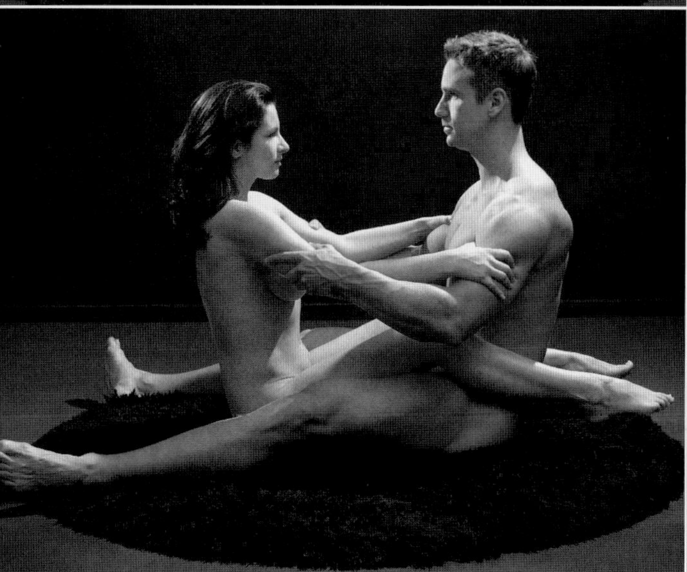

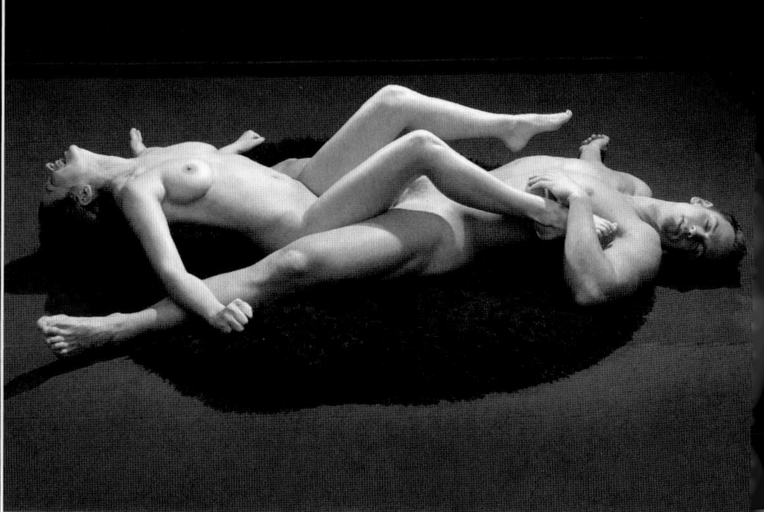

c

d

The Open-Eyed Partner Clench and Hold ▲

- **a** Sit, gaze, and breathe.
- **b** Rock and add Kegels.
- **c** Clench, hold, and let go.
- **d** Fall backward and enjoy the afterglow. (See full explanation on page 123.)

or speak to him. He will unconsciously receive this belief. This will support him in creating these things for himself. Remember, focus on the goal, not the pro-cess. When you see your friend sitting comfortably in chemotherapy, you are still holding a vision of illness. Instead, see him cancer-free, in robust health, and enjoying a Hawaiian vacation.

Here are just a few of the ways that you can use sex magic to aid yourself and others.

SEX MAGIC FOR YOURSELF

- To change unwanted habits and old behaviors;
- To relieve stress;
- To relieve menstrual cramps, back pain, and headaches;
- To relieve jet lag;
- To relieve pain and fear;
- To improve a relationship;
- To improve business;
- To get a job or a promotion;
- To make more money;
- To soothe painful emotions;
- To receive information or guidance about a problem.

SEX MAGIC FOR OTHERS

- To send pain relief or healing;
- To send guidance;
- To send peace and tranquility;
- To say thank you for a gift or for assistance;
- To say happy birthday or happy anniversary;
- To send support in handling a loss;
- To send congratulations on hearing of a friend's good fortune;
- To contact a friend who has been out of touch;
- To end the AIDS crisis (or cancer, heart disease, etc.);
- To support a world leader who is working on behalf of peace and justice;
- To support a change of attitude in a world leader you do not feel is doing the right thing.

Practicing sex magic with a partner is a particularly delicious and powerful way to raise twice the energy of a solo sex-magic ritual. You and your partner can hold the same vision or different ones. You can raise sexual energy any way you like—intercourse, oral sex, breath, movement, sight, sound, erotic massage—it all works. I especially like the quality and quantity of sexual energy raised in a partnered version of the Clench and Hold that you practiced in chapter 2. In addition to providing a full-body orgasmic experience, it is great practice for learning to keep your eyes open during all sorts of orgasms.

THE OPEN-EYED PARTNER CLENCH AND HOLD

Sit facing your partner. Gaze into his or her eyes. Breathe together using the Heart Breath (see chapter 2). Relax your jaw and face, open the back of your throat, and breathe in through your mouth, gently but fully. Exhale. Don't push the breath out; just let it fall out of your body. Take in as much air as you can as effortlessly as you can, then let it go. Rock back and forth and add Kegels. Breathe and rock with the intention of building as much energy as possible—really go for it! As the energy builds, breathe in fuller and faster breaths. When you both feel so inclined, take in a deep breath together and hold it. Gaze into each other's eyes as you clench and hold your buttocks, abdominal and PC muscles. After about fifteen seconds, let go. Keep your eyes open and look into your partner's eyes. Now you have a choice: You can either fall backward and away from each other, close your eyes, and enjoy the afterglow, or you can begin breathing again and go for another Clench and Hold. Try a sequence of two or three or more rounds of breathing and clenching and holding.

The sitting open-eyed Clench and Hold is a powerful way to raise a lot of orgasmic energy with or without sex magic. If you are doing sex magic, visualize your shared or separate desires before you start breathing. Then let go of your vision. Concentrate only on breathing, eye gazing, rocking back and forth, and raising lots of energy. When you eventually clench your muscles and hold your breath, flash your vision on your mind's

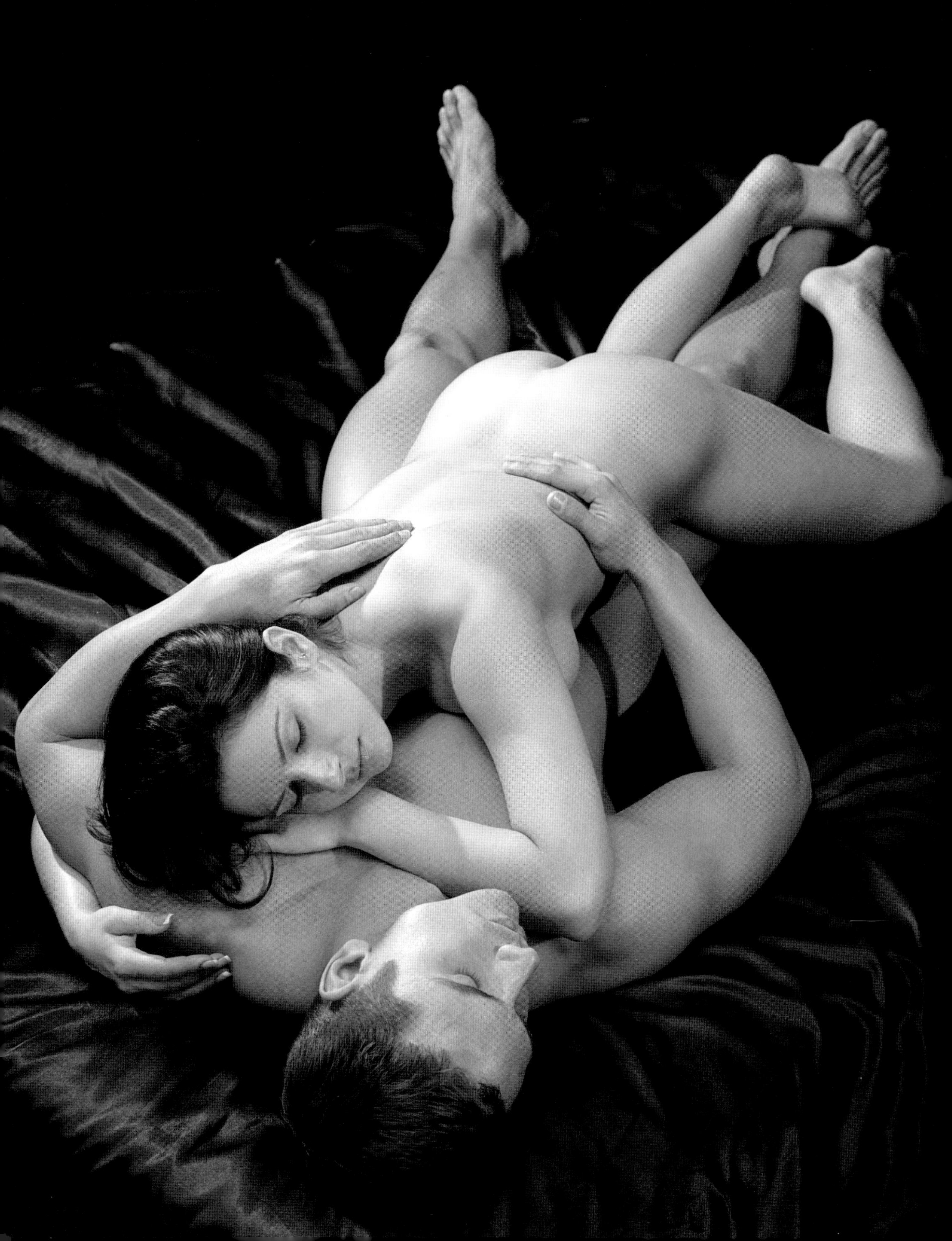

eye as you look into your partner's eyes. I like to imagine my partner's eyes as magnification mirrors that magnify my vision a thousand times and reflect it out into the universe to work its magic.

Dedicate Your Magic to Your Relationship

One of the most magical aspects of sex is the magic within a sexual relationship. Whether your relationship is full-time, part-time, or exists only for the joint exploration of sexual mysteries, there is a rhythm and a dance to sex that temporarily turns two people into one. While you and your lover each experience yourself from within yourself, your separateness eventually merges into mutual participation as a single, larger reality. This boundaryless, egoless, everywhere-and-nowhere space is ideal for exploring the new possibilities for your relationship.

The next time you make love, dedicate your sexual energy to the expansion of your relationship. What are the things you like about your relationship? What is vitally important to you? What delights you? What are you willing to overlook? What makes you crazy? What would you like to change? Our relationships are constantly changing and growing whether we like it or not. A relationship is like a garden. If it is not tended to, it will grow as many weeds as flowers, and eventually the weeds will push the flowers out of the garden altogether. When we take a relationship for granted and just let it meander along haphazardly, it may grow and change in unpleasant and unkind ways. In order to have a relationship as intuitive, insightful, brilliant, and passionate as you would like it to be, you and your partner must continually commit and recommit to it. This allows the mutual discovery of a magical, intimate place filled with both freedom and security.

In order to direct sex magic to your specific relationship goals, you first need to know what they are. Try to devote one day a month exclusively to your partner and your relationship. During your quiet and leisurely start to this day, take a pencil and paper and list your values. Values are not priorities. Priorities are things you do. Values are why you do them. Some of your values may be freedom, personal growth, prosperity, security, service to others, pleasure, beauty, commitment to career, physical fitness, or loyalty to family. Rank your values from most important to least important. Now share these values with your partner, notice which you share and which you don't. You do not have to hold the same values as your partner, but it is important for each of you to know what the other's values are. If, for example, your highest value right now is personal growth, then you're going to prioritize taking a workshop over going skiing. If your partner's most important value right now is physical fitness, he would rather go skiing. When you know each other's values, it is easy for him to schedule his skiing trip for the same weekend you'll be at the workshop. No hurt feelings, no unconscious resentments. Once you have your values in place, you can make agreements. What do you want and need from each other? How can you support each other in having what you both want? When you have your values and your agreements, you can use sex magic to enrich these parts of your relationship. This practical, positive way of relating mindfully requires a commitment from both partners to approach their relationship as a tool for expansion of consciousness, for growth, and for imagining new possibilities. The rewards of that commitment are a vibrant and loving relationship filled with magic, insight, brilliance, and a passion for life at its best.

ACKNOWLEDGMENTS

MY HEARTFELT GRATITUDE TO:

Allan Penn, for his inspired erotic photography, which has expressed my vision for this book perfectly.

Catherine Carter, Hayley Caspers, Dan and Dawn, Kutira Decosterd, Betty Dodson, Bridgett Harrington, Louise L. Hay, Jwala, Joseph Kramer, Chester Mainard, Mark and Patricia Michaels, Linda Montano, Dr. Jonn Mumford, Jenny Navaro and Steve Cairnduff, Judith Orloff, Osho, David and Ellen Ramsdale, Sir Andrew, Annie Sprinkle, and Kenneth Ray Stubbs, for inspiring me with their passion, wisdom, and erotic mischief.

Bianca and Steve, for being so talented and such good sports.

Holly Schmidt, Rosalind Wanke, Alexis Sullivan, Arlene Bouras, and, most especially, my editrix extraordinaire, Wendy Gardner, for a delightful publishing experience.

Kate Bornstein, my partner in life, love, and art, for her invaluable editing and her unwavering love and support.

P. Kitty for her delight in the writing process.

ABOUT THE AUTHOR

BARBARA CARRELLAS IS THE FOUNDER OF Urban Tantra, an approach to sacred Sexuality that adapts and blends conscious sexuality practices from Tanra to S/M, and the cofounder of Erotic Awakening, a pioneering series of workshops focusing on the physical, spiritual, and healing powers of sex. Barbara was named Best Tantric Sex Seminar Leader in New York City by *Time Out* magazine for her Urban Tantra workshops. She is the author of two books, numerous articles and essays, and an audio series called, *The Pleasure Principle*. Her Web site can be found at www.barbaracarrellas.com

OTHER HOT BOOKS FROM QUIVER

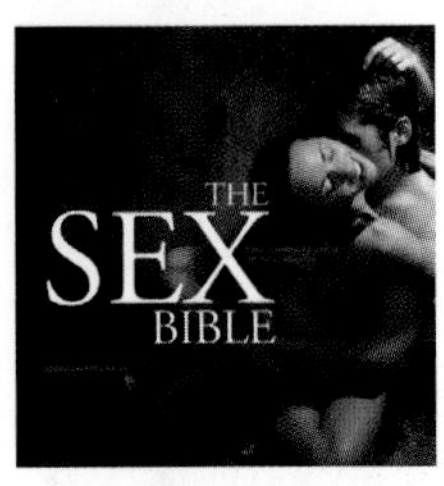

The Sex Bible
The Complete Guide to Sexual Love
By Susan Crain Bakos
ISBN-13: 978-1-59233-227-4
ISBN-10: 1-59233-227-7
$30.00/£19.99/$38.95 CAN

The Sex Bible is an authoritative, comprehensive, and beautifully photographed sex resource book that provides in-depth treatment of sexual topics in frank detail. The book is arranged into different sections, including "Foreplay," "Sex Toys," and "Oral Sex." It explores sexual subjects you are either familiar with, or until now, never even knew existed. Couples will be captivated by personal anecdotes interspersed throughout. Illustrated with full-color photography, *The Sex Bible* will not only educate couples, but also it will help heighten sexual enjoyment.

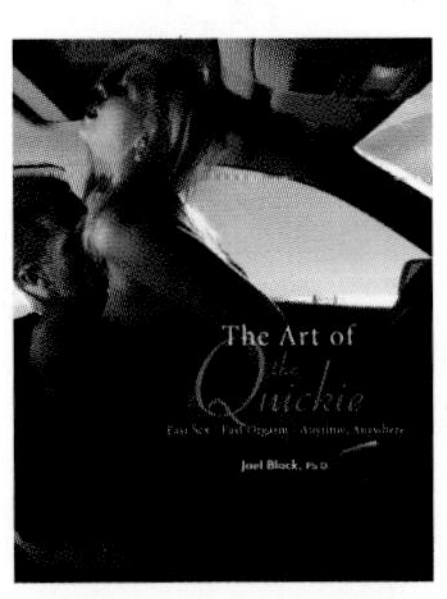

The Art of the Quickie
Fast Sex, Fast Orgasm, Anytime, Anywhere
By Joel D. Block, Ph.D.
ISBN-13: 978-1-59233-240-3
ISBN-10: 1-59233-240-4
$19.99/£12.99/$25.95 CAN

The Art of the Quickie will coach readers how to have quick, but rewarding sex. Quickies can be even more fulfilling as those long sessions because the thrill involved in having sex unexpectedly or in forbidden locations adds a potent element of excitement. But what about women, is the quickie fair to them? *The Art of the Quickie* features definitive guidelines for women to experience faster orgasms—in 5 minutes!—thereby relieving men of the performance anxiety that often accompanies the responsibility of bringing their partners to orgasm.

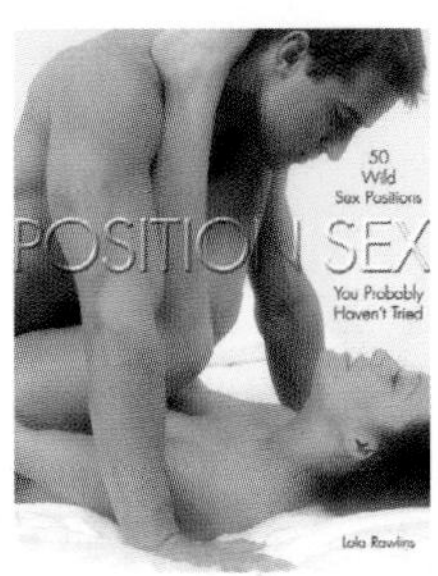

Position seX
50 Wild Sex Positions You Probably Haven't Tried
By Lola Rawlins
ISBN-13: 978-1-59233-238-0
ISBN-10: 1-59233-238-2
$19.99/£12.99/$25.95 CAN

For couples who might be stuck in a one-position nooky rut, *Position seX* instructs couples on how to spice up their sex life and be more adventurous in the bedroom (or any room, counter, or chair in the house.) The book features full-color photographs of each hot, new position, as well as slight acrobatic variations on good old standbys, such as the missionary position. In addition to new positions, *Position seX* also provides tips on sexual accoutrements —dildoes, vibrators, sexy lingerie, and lubricants—to further spice up your fun.